Quality
in family practice
Book of Tools

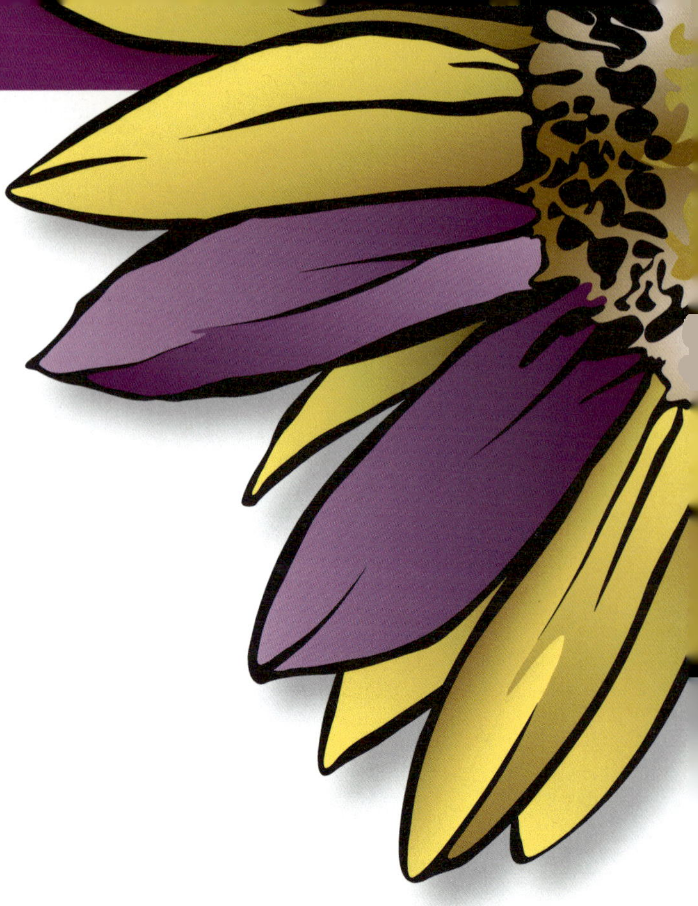

Authors: **Cheryl Levitt and Linda Hilts**

***Quality* Book of Tools**

ISBN 978-1-926633-38-1

Book design by Côté Design, Toronto

For permission to use any content of the *Quality* Book of Tools, please contact Dr Cheryl Levitt at the **Department of Family Medicine**, McMaster University, 100 Main Street West,
MHC, 5th Floor, Hamilton, ON, Canada. L8P1H6
Tel: (905) 525-9140 x 28500 Fax: (905) 527-4440 email: clevitt@mcmaster.ca

Recommended Citation:
Levitt C, Hilts L. *Quality* Book of Tools. Hamilton: McMaster Innovation Press; 2010.

Links updated October 2015.
Previous links updated: June 2011, November 2012, June 2013, and August 2014.

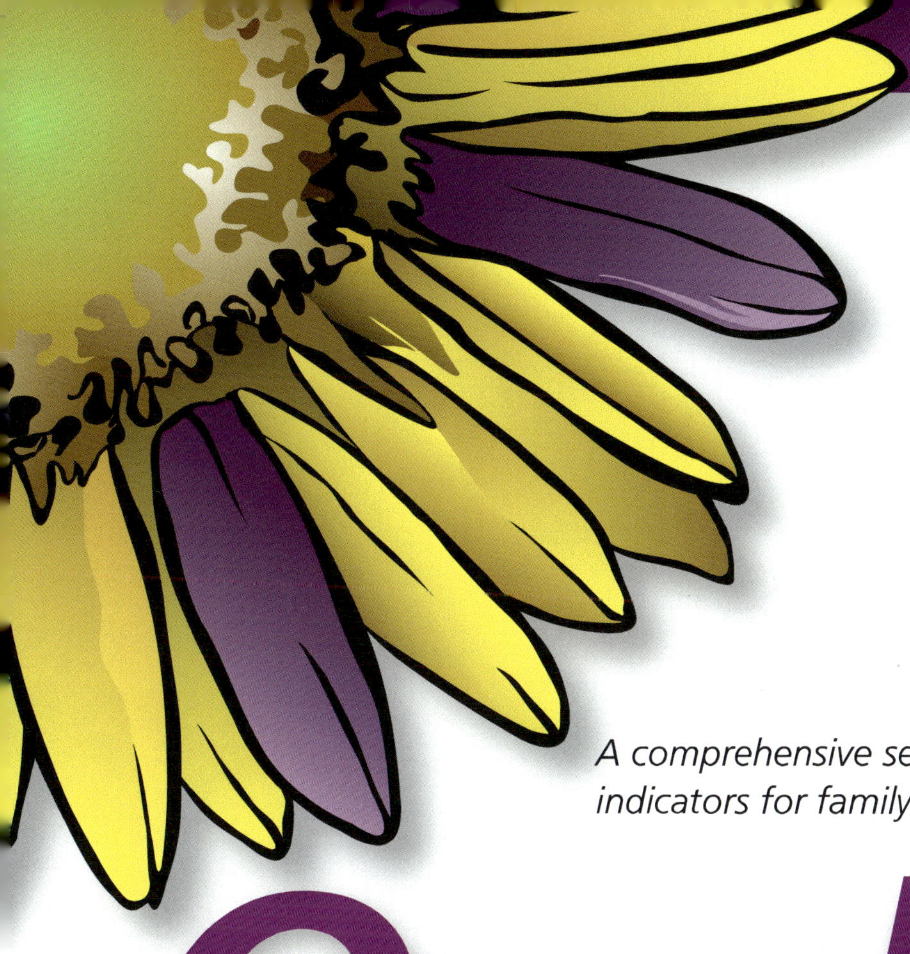

A comprehensive set of quality performance indicators for family practices.

Quality
in family practice
Book of Tools

Cheryl Levitt MBBCh CCFP FCFP
Professor, Department of Family Medicine, McMaster University

Linda Hilts RN BScN MEd
Assistant Professor, Department of Family Medicine, McMaster University

McMaster Innovation Press, Hamilton, Canada

TABLE OF CONTENTS

Dedication

This *Quality* Book of Tools is dedicated to all the family physicians and primary care providers committed to continuously improving how they provide care for their patients.

Acknowledgements

Quality Book of Tools Review Team

David Price MD, CCFP, FCFP,
Associate Professor,
Department of Family Medicine,
McMaster University, Hamilton,
Ontario, Canada

Lisa Dolovich,
BScPhm, MSc, PharmD,
Associate Professor,
Department of Family Medicine,
McMaster University, Hamilton,
Ontario, Canada

Jan Kasperski RN, MHSc, CHE
Chief Executive Officer,
Ontario College of Family Physicians,
Toronto, Ontario, Canada

Jennifer McGregor,
B.Comm., RD, CDE
Registered Dietitian/
Certified Diabetes Educator
St. Catharines, Ontario, Canada

Carol Lane
Administrative Assistant

Wendy Chin
Quality Project Manager, 2008-2010

Betty Ho
Quality Book Manager, 2010

Xiaoke Katherine Li
Research Assistant, 2010
McMaster University, Hamilton,
Ontario, Canada

Ontario Ministry of Health and Long Term Care (MOHLTC)

We would like to acknowledge the Ontario MOHLTC for providing funding for the early development and testing of the Quality in Family Practice Assessment Tool

International & National Indicators/Tools

We would like to acknowledge the beneficial influence of the following International Tools in the development of the *Quality* Book of Tools:

Royal New Zealand College of General Practitioners. Aiming for Excellence – An Assessment Tool for New Zealand General Practice. 3rd ed [monograph online]. New Zealand: Royal New Zealand College of General Practitioners (RNZCGP); 2009 [cited 2010 Jul 21]. Available from: **www.rnzcgp.org.nz/assets/documents/CORNERSTONE/Aiming-for-Excellence-2009-including-record-review.pdf**

Royal Australian College of General Practitioners National Expert Committee on Standards for General Practices. Standards for General Practices. 3rd ed [monograph online]. South Melbourne: The Royal Australian College of General Practitioners (RACGP); Updated edition available from: **www.racgp.org.au/your-practice/standards/** 2013 May [cited 2014 Jul 17].

TOPAS-Europe. European Practice Assessment (EPA) – Easy to use and scientifically developed quality management for general practice [Internet]. 2008 Jan 9 [cited 2015 May 19]. Available from: **www.equip.ch/files/31/epa_information_paper_english_vs11.pdf**

NHS Employers & General Practitioners Committee (BMA). Quality and Outcomes Framework – Guidance for GMS contract 2009/10 [Internet]. 2009 Mar [cited 2014 Jul 09].
Available from: **www.google.ca/url?sa=t&rct=j&q=&esrc=s&source=web&cd=3&ved=0CCoQFjAC&url=http%3A%2F%2Fwww.networks.nhs.uk%2Fnhs-networks%2Flondon-qof-network%2Fdocuments%2FQOF%2520Guidance%2520The%2520Green%2520Document%25202009-2010_Final.pdf%2Fat_download%2Ffile&ei=az-jU67wKtaLqAaT3oLADg&usg=AFQjCNGtxmeUjceWod7xoucptgXpFtpjBQ&bvm=bv.69411363,d.b2k**

Canadian Institute for Health Information. Pan-Canadian Primary Health Care Indicators [monograph online]. Ottawa: Canadian Institute for Health Information; 2006 [cited 2014 Jul 09].
Available from: **www.cihi.ca/CIHI-ext-portal/pdf/internet/PDF_PHC_INDI_REPORT1VOL1FIN_EN**
https://secure.cihi.ca/free_products/PHC_Indicator_Report_1-Volume_2_Final_E.pdf

Cheryl Levitt MBBCh CCFP FCFP
Professor, Department of Family Medicine, McMaster University, Hamilton, Ontario, Canada

Cheryl Levitt is a family physician and a professor in the Department of Family Medicine at McMaster University. She was born in South Africa, trained at the University of the Witwatersrand in Johannesburg and interned at Baragwanath Hospital, Soweto. Cheryl practiced rurally in British Columbia for 7 years and has been an academic family physician at McGill and McMaster Universities since 1984. She was Chair of the Department of Family Medicine at McMaster University from 1996-2006, President of the Ontario College of Family Physicians from 2005-2006 and is presently the Senior Research Advisor for the College of Family Physicians of Canada. She led the Quality in Family Practice project from 2000-2009. Cheryl has published widely on primary care issues, medical migration of foreign doctors, gender equity and maternal and child health. She has received a number of awards including the Individual National Breastfeeding Seminar Award of Excellence in 1999, the South African Women for Women HEALTH Award in 2004, the Enid Johnson Award from the Federation of Medical Women of Canada in 2008, the Wonca (World Organization of Family Doctors) Fellowship Award in 2010, the Jean Pierre Depins Award of the College of Family Physicians of Canada in 2010, and the YWCA Woman of Distinction Award for Health Wellness for the City of Hamilton in 2011.

Linda Hilts RN BScN MEd
Assistant Professor, School of Nursing
Associate Member, Department of Family Medicine, McMaster University, Hamilton, Ontario, Canada

Linda Hilts started her nursing career as an operating room nurse in cardiovascular surgery at Hamilton General Hospital. She worked part-time in rehabilitation medicine with stroke and spinal cord patients at Holbrook, Chedoke Hospital, before joining VON and later CCAC. After completing a BScN from McMaster and then a MEd from Brock University, Linda worked at the Hamilton Civic Hospitals in a newly created position of patient education coordinator. She started working for Stonechurch Family Health Centre in 1998 as a family practice nurse and became involved in resident education, becoming the education coordinator for Stonechurch and then FHT coordinator. Linda has been the nursing consultant for the Quality in Family Practice program since 2002. Linda has won a number of awards for her work in primary care, including the Sibley Award for part-time faculty at McMaster University and the Ted Evans Scholarship Award for exemplary practice in the four principles of family medicine. Since retiring from full-time work in 2009, she has continued to work as a primary care consultant with a focus on OSCAR clinical training and improving quality in primary care settings through the Quality in Family Practice program.

This *Quality* Book of Tools has been evolving in Ontario, Canada, over the past ten years. In 2000, Dr. Ronald MacVicar, a general practitioner from Inverness in Scotland, offered to help us develop a tool for assessing quality in family practice as part of his sabbatical at McMaster University in Hamilton. Working with local family doctors, we developed an early version called the Hamilton Tool. It was based on the Scottish Quality Practice Awards, which was a well-established program in Scotland. We added some additional indicators to make it more applicable to Hamilton. In 2003, we, at McMaster University, partnered with the Ontario College of Family Physicians, to obtain funding from the Ontario MOHLTC to develop a Quality tool that could be used in family practices throughout Ontario. Adopting elements from New Zealand and Australia, we drafted a tool to test in the Quality in Family Practice program (a voluntary quality assessment program – for more information see **www.qualityinfamilypractice.com)** in a variety of family practices, in two phases, in 2005 and 2007. In 2008-2009, we undertook an international review of primary care quality-assessment tools and a modified Delphi process with Canadian experts to validate the indicators we had drafted. Over the past year, we have rewritten, refined and categorized the indicators to align with the work being done in quality at the Ontario Health Quality Council and the Institute of Medicine in the United States.

This is the first edition of the *Quality* Book of Tools. It will continue to evolve as the work progresses and as we discover better ways to measure and assess the quality of family practices in Ontario.

The *Quality* Book of Tools is intended to help family doctors and other primary care providers, teachers, researchers and decision makers assess and evaluate the complex nature of primary care. The Tool allows users to categorize the activities of family practices into practice management and clinical effectiveness. The intention is that family practices will use the indicators to facilitate the measurement of performance in family practices, both practice management and clinical.

The Introduction to the *Quality* Book of Tools includes some details of the history of the Tool's development and guidance on how to use it. Each of the eight chapters that follow comprises a category, with indicators and criteria specific to a particular part of the practice. Further information, in the form of links to key sites, is provided to help guide the development of improvement processes based on best practices. The up to date links have been collected in a resource database that can be found at **http://quality.resources.machealth.ca**.

None of this would have been possible without the administrative skills of Carol Lane, Wendy Chin, Katherine Li and Betty Ho whom we want to thank for helping us convert a messy manuscript into this publication. Thanks also to David Price, Lisa Dolovich, Jan Kasperski and Jennifer McGregor, for reviewing the manuscript and providing helpful suggestions and Dr. Anthony Levinson for creating the resource database. We are grateful to the Department of Family Medicine at McMaster University and the Ontario College of Family Physicians for their ongoing support of this project.

Cheryl Levitt & Linda Hilts
Hamilton, Ontario, November 2010

2003-2009 *QUALITY* TOOL CONTRIBUTORS

Project Management Team

Cheryl Levitt, Project Lead

David Price, Physician Consultant

Linda Hilts, Nursing Consultant

Jan Kasperski, OCFP Representative

Project Team Members

Angela Barbara, Project Manager & Researcher

Jamie Baxter, Website Design

Eileen Hanna, Project Manager

Phyllis Jansen, Research Coordinator

Colin McMullan, Research Coordinator

Tammy Villeneuve, Administrative Assistant

Steering Committee Members

Jack Azulay, Patient Representative

Anne Barber, Nurse Practitioner Representative

Elizabeth Beader, Executive Director of North Hamilton Community Health Centre

Janie Bowles-Jordan, Pharmacist Representative

Lisa Dolovich, Pharmacist Representative

Jennifer Frid, Receptionist Consultant

Carol Hayter, Patient Representative

Michelle Martin, Patient Representative

Jennifer McGregor, Dietitian Representative

Ruth Morris, Family Physician Consultant

Mari Rainer, Receptionist Representative

Carol Ridge, Manager Representative

David Smith, Social Worker Representative

Refining the Quality Assessment Tool and modified Delphi Project

Lisa Dolovich, Principal Investigator

Cheryl Levitt, Principal Investigator

David Price, Principal Investigator

Kalpana Nair, Project Manager & Researcher

Consultants

Alan Abelsohn, Consultant on Tool Development

David Chan, IT Consultant

Michael Mills, Australian & New Zealand Site Visitor

Cathy Whyte, Cost Analysis

Chris Woodward, Research Consultant

Corresponding Consultants

Maureen Gillon, New Zealand

Bruce Bagley, United States

Rachelle Vial, United Kingdom

Ronald MacVicar, Scotland

Jim DuRose, New Zealand

INTRODUCTION

Overview

The *Quality* Book of Tools is a comprehensive book of practice management and clinical care indicators for improving quality in primary care, family practice settings in Ontario, Canada. This *Quality* Book of Tools 2010 was developed following an international review and modified Delphi process in 2008-2009 and is the revised version of the 2003-2005 *Quality in Family Practice Tool*. It is available as a hard copy book and in an open source, web-based version. It is designed for family practices in Ontario but could be useful to primary care settings throughout Canada and internationally.

This *Quality* Book of Tools includes a conceptual framework of categories and values depicted in the *Quality* Flower, a yellow and purple sunflower chosen as a metaphor for the Book of Tools.

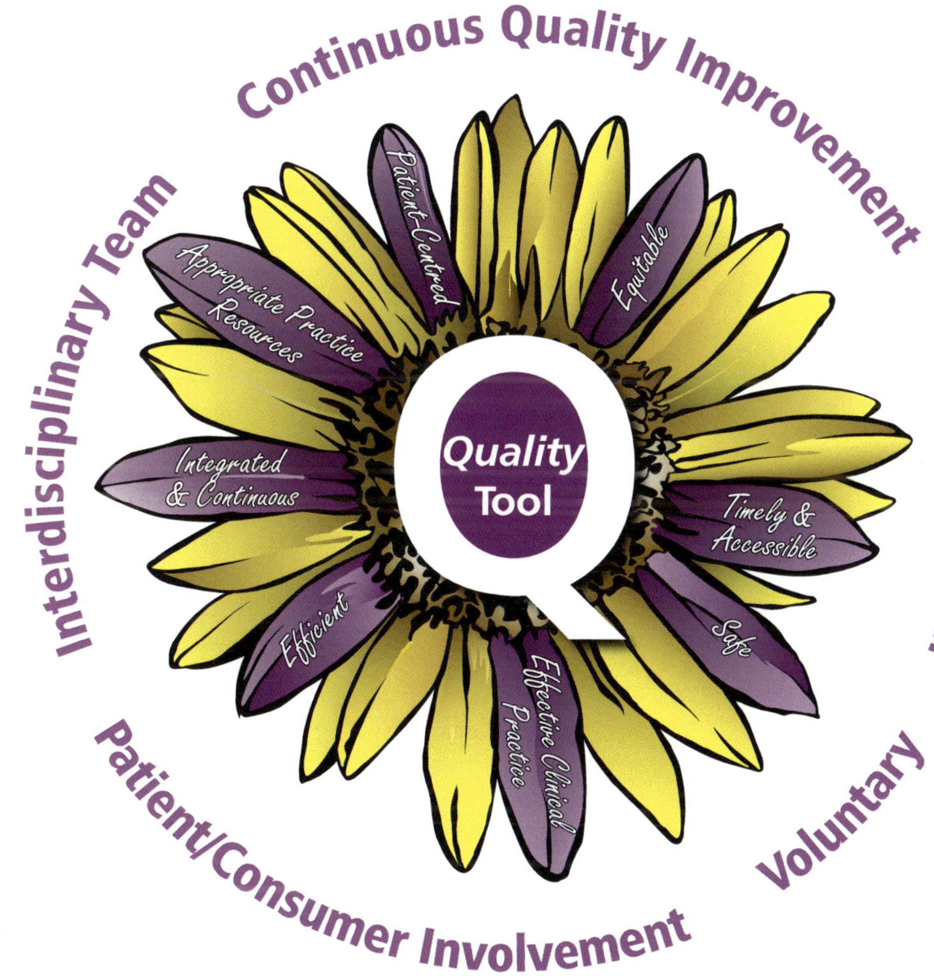

OVERVIEW

Just as a sunflower follows the sun throughout the day and grows vigorously under its rays, but withers without water and sunshine, *Quality* in primary care requires attention, nurturing and support to flourish. The future of the sunflower lies in its centre, just as the practice team's commitment to continuous quality improvement is at the heart of *Quality*. The petals of the sunflower represent the categories of indicators of quality in a family practice setting. Eight categories have been identified in this 1st Edition *Quality* Book of Tools, and in the future more may be added as primary care evolves and quality improvements develop further. (The sunflower's yellow petals represent as-yet unidentified categories.) Purple was chosen as the colour of *Quality* because it is a complex and unique hue that stands alone, representing the complex nature of quality and the challenge of including continuous improvement in the normal rhythm of everyday work. However, with time and experience, the inherent value and rewards of incorporating *Quality* into day-to-day activities become ever clearer.

The five values integral to developing a sustainable quality-improvement culture in primary care in Ontario, in no particular order, are:

- A culture of **continuous quality improvement** (CQI) that is never-ending and included in usual daily activity. The Plan-Do-Study-Act (PDSA) cycles for testing a change can be used to apply CQI.
- A process of **self-reflection** that allows the family practice to undertake actions needed to assess its current standing in terms of best practices.
- Making such assessments in a **voluntary**, non-threatening manner.
- The inclusion of **patient/consumer** involvement.
- **Interdisciplinary team** development and functioning.

The five values surround the *Quality* flower, which has eight petals representing the eight categories that incorporate the common elements of family practice activities. These eight categories also align with the established aims of the Institute of Medicine: Crossing the Quality Chasm and the Ontario Health Quality Council's Reporting Framework: Attributes of a High Performing Health System[1,2] (Table 1). The eight Categories are in no particular order and are labelled for convenience:

A Patient-Centred

B Equitable

C Timely and Accessible

D Safe

E Effective Clinical Practice

F Efficient

G Integrated and Continuous

H Appropriate Practice Resources

The eight Categories have 34 Sub-Categories, which group similar Indicators together. The Sub-Categories have 70 Indicators, which can be separated into 43 practice management and 27 clinical indicators. The indicators have been systematically designed to identify the common elements of family practice performance that can be assessed to improve the quality of care. Even so, the list of indicators is not exhaustive and may not include all of the elements that are important and relevant for individual practices. Each indicator has Criteria that can be counted or measured in order to assess quality of performance of an indicator. Criteria are discrete, definable, measurable and explicit. There are three types of criteria:

- ⚖ **Legal and Safety** – required by law*
- ★ **Essential** – required to demonstrate best practice
- ❊ **Desirable** – required to demonstrate additional quality

*(*Assumptions about ⚖ indicators are based on the nature of these indicators and the regulations that qualify them)*

It is expected that most family practices will first meet the requirements for the legal and essential criteria, and then strive to meet the desirable criteria.

Best-practice guidelines and the associated audit requirements are extremely complex and require external and internal resources which are not universally available in family practices in Ontario at time of writing. Although these guidelines reflect best practice, few practices meet all the criteria outlined in the *Quality* Book of Tools for monitoring quality performance. Best practice will need to evolve and be updated over time. The indicators and criteria in the book are not intended to be considered standard of practice in Ontario. They are intended as a guide only, and, in the spirit of continuous quality improvement (CQI) and rapid cycle change, to assist practices to make choices. Some indicators may take priority over others, but over time all the indicators in a family practice would be incorporated and be part of an ongoing quality improvement program.

The *Quality* Tool is a web-based instrument. Each indicator has a section called *Further Information* that lists relevant web links, which can be accessed directly from the electronic version. The up to date links have been collected in a resource database that can be found at **http://quality.resources.machealth.ca**. Each criterion is qualified by the *Interpretation* which explains the expected performance measurement activities that must be completed to meet the requirements of the criterion. These *Further Information* links connect to helpful on-line resources in Ontario or elsewhere (for example, government sites, professional organizations' sites and best-practice guidelines as of 2010, such as the Cochrane Library review, and so on). The authors are not responsible for and do not necessarily endorse the content on the linked websites.

Background

The *Quality* Book of Tools is a key feature of the Quality program for voluntary assessment by trained peer assessors in family practices in Ontario. The Quality program team (a collaborative group from McMaster University and the Ontario College of Family Physicians), funded by the Ontario Ministry of Health and Long-Term Care since 2003, developed and tested the program and the original Quality Tool in a number of phases. In 2003-2005, the team reviewed the national and international literature on quality assessments in family practice/primary care, conducted focus-group interviews, environmental scans and teleconferences with patients and practitioners, and visited sites in the United Kingdom, Australia, New Zealand and Toronto, Canada that operate quality programs. The information guided the process for the Quality program and tool development. The project team was assisted by a steering committee composed of primary care providers, administrative staff and patients/consumers, a number of consultants and an advisory committee of key stakeholders. The program and tool was tested in three practices in urban and rural settings in Ontario in 2005-2006, and in seven family health teams (including 130 health-care providers caring for 74,000 patients) in 2007-2008. A modified Delphi process, conducted in 2008-2009 on the Indicators, led to a complete rewrite of the Quality Tool in 2009-2010. The revised version is called The *Quality* Book of Tools and covers the complex scope of family practice.

Why have a *Quality* Book of Tools?

Family physicians and other primary care providers generally strive to deliver quality care to their patients. Assessment is essential to evaluate the level of quality, and an organized tool allows practices to list and rank the crucial components that comprise quality care. The *Quality* Book of Tools is a comprehensive guide that builds on local, national and international experiences, is validated through a panel of experts and is written by and for primary care providers in Ontario. This tool can be used on its own or as an essential component of the voluntary assessment program *Quality in Family Practice* in Ontario. Practitioners and practices might be motivated to use the tool for several reasons: proactively to assess the quality of care or reactively to fix an identified problem.

Where to find the *Quality* Book of Tools?

The *Quality* Book of Tools is designed to be accessible and available to practices through **www.qualitybookoftools.ca** as a web book and can be purchased through McMASTER INNOVATION PRESS as a print-on-demand "library-quality book". The whole book or each chapter can be read or printed as needed from the website.

Continuous Quality Improvement

The *Quality* Book of Tools is best used with a continuous quality improvement (CQI) approach. CQI is the process of collecting data about a particular practice or service to benchmark performance, tracking and validating indicators that affect outcomes, and recognizing problems in processes of care and practice management. CQI is a culture of never-ending improvement of the whole system as part of normal daily activity, continually striving to act according to the best available knowledge. The assumption behind quality measurement is that unless we learn something about what we are doing, we are unlikely to know that it needs improving or how to improve it. Measurement alone, however, is not useful – it must be associated with a CQI approach.

A number of models and cycles can be used to apply CQI on an ongoing basis. One of the most commonly used approaches that has been successful in family practice settings is the Plan-Do-Study-Act (PDSA) cycle.

PDSA enables testing of changes on a small scale to determine if they are beneficial. Each small improvement builds knowledge and confidence and enables continued reflection on the quality of the practice.

PDSA

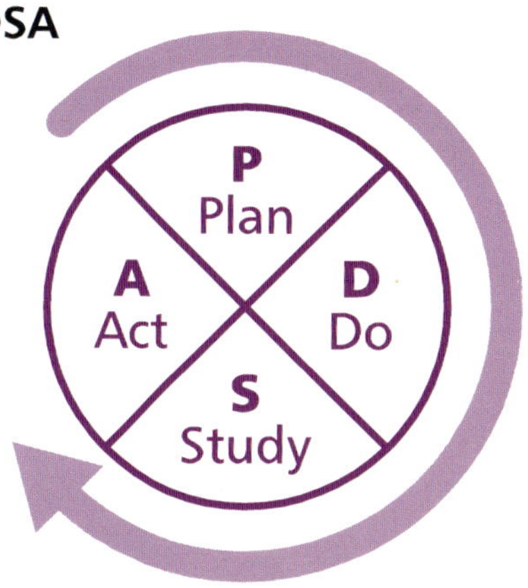

Plan Develop a plan for improving quality

Do Execute the plan, first on a small scale

Study Evaluate feedback to confirm or to adjust the plan

Act Make the plan permanent or study the adjustments

Don Berwick[3]

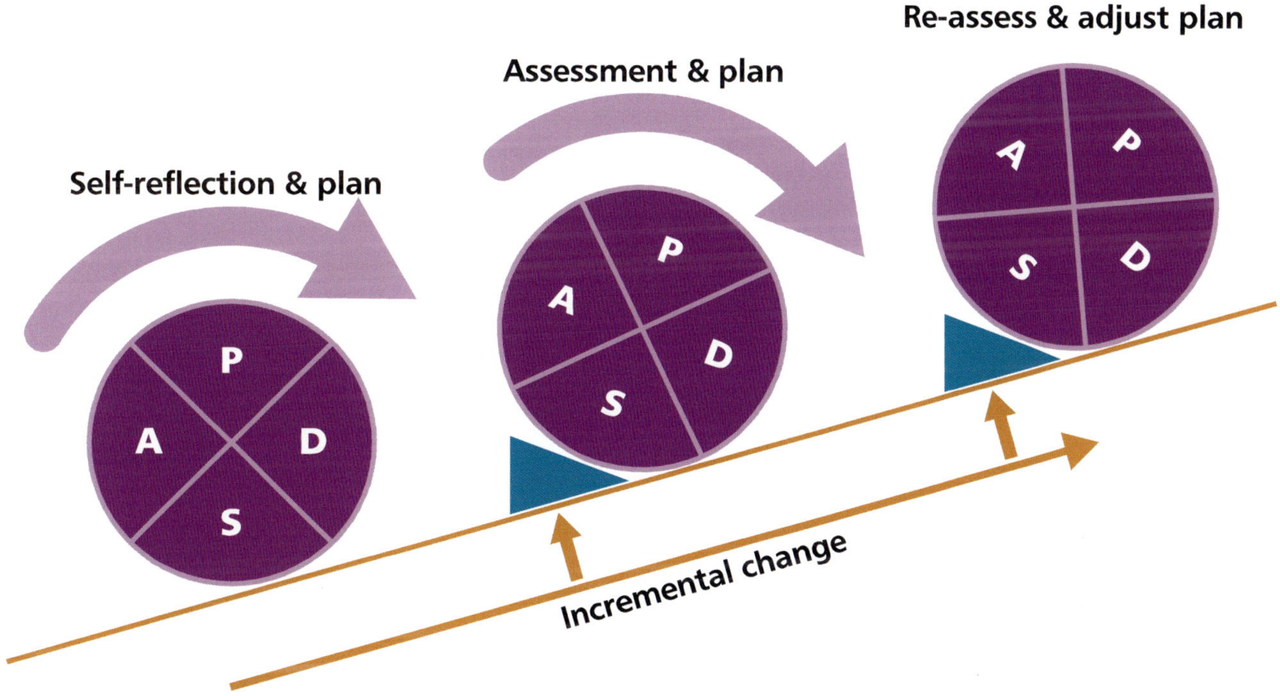

Institute for Healthcare Improvement[4]

How to use the *Quality* Book of Tools

> **"The journey of a thousand miles begins with one step." Lao Tzu**

The *Quality* Book of Tools provides a set of indicators and criteria that help the practice reflect on its strengths as well as areas that need improvement ("where you are"). The practice can then focus on actions that over time will achieve that improvement ("where you want to be").

The *Quality* Book of Tools is large and its scope ambitious. It can be intimidating, so here are our suggestions for getting started:

- The book is a compendium of common primary care best practices. It is designed to be used to improve the whole practice, but you can begin that process with a single indicator, ideally in a voluntary assessment program such as the *Quality in Family Practice* program.
- Read the introduction to get an overview of the purpose of the book and the different Categories, Sub-Categories, Indicators and Criteria. (Category D: Safe, for example, covers such things as cold chain, infection control, drug management and record-keeping). The book is divided into eight Categories with 34 Sub-Categories and 70 Indicators. Each indicator links to evidence-based websites under the heading *Further Information*. The up to date links have been collected in a resource database that can be found at **http://quality.resources.machealth.ca**
- Read and reflect on CQI and how to use PDSA cycles to improve quality in your practice.
- Decide which areas of your practice you would like to improve and in what order. Do you want to assess the whole practice or just certain aspects? Even if you intend to assess the entire practice, you can begin with one area, such as practice management or clinical care.
- Choose a category and drill down to a sub-category. Once you have decided where you want to focus your attention, start with the indicator most relevant to your practice and review the criteria.
- Then determine whether you meet the *Interpretation*. Many practices will find they already meet the requirements for some indicators and criteria.
- Apply a PDSA approach to any criterion the practice does not meet. Assess where you are and what improvements are needed. Plan the first step needed to get where you want to go. Do that activity, then measure and evaluate whether you have accomplished what you wanted to achieve. If not, repeat the PDSA cycle. Sometimes more than one activity needs to be done before the *Interpretation* for a criterion can be met.

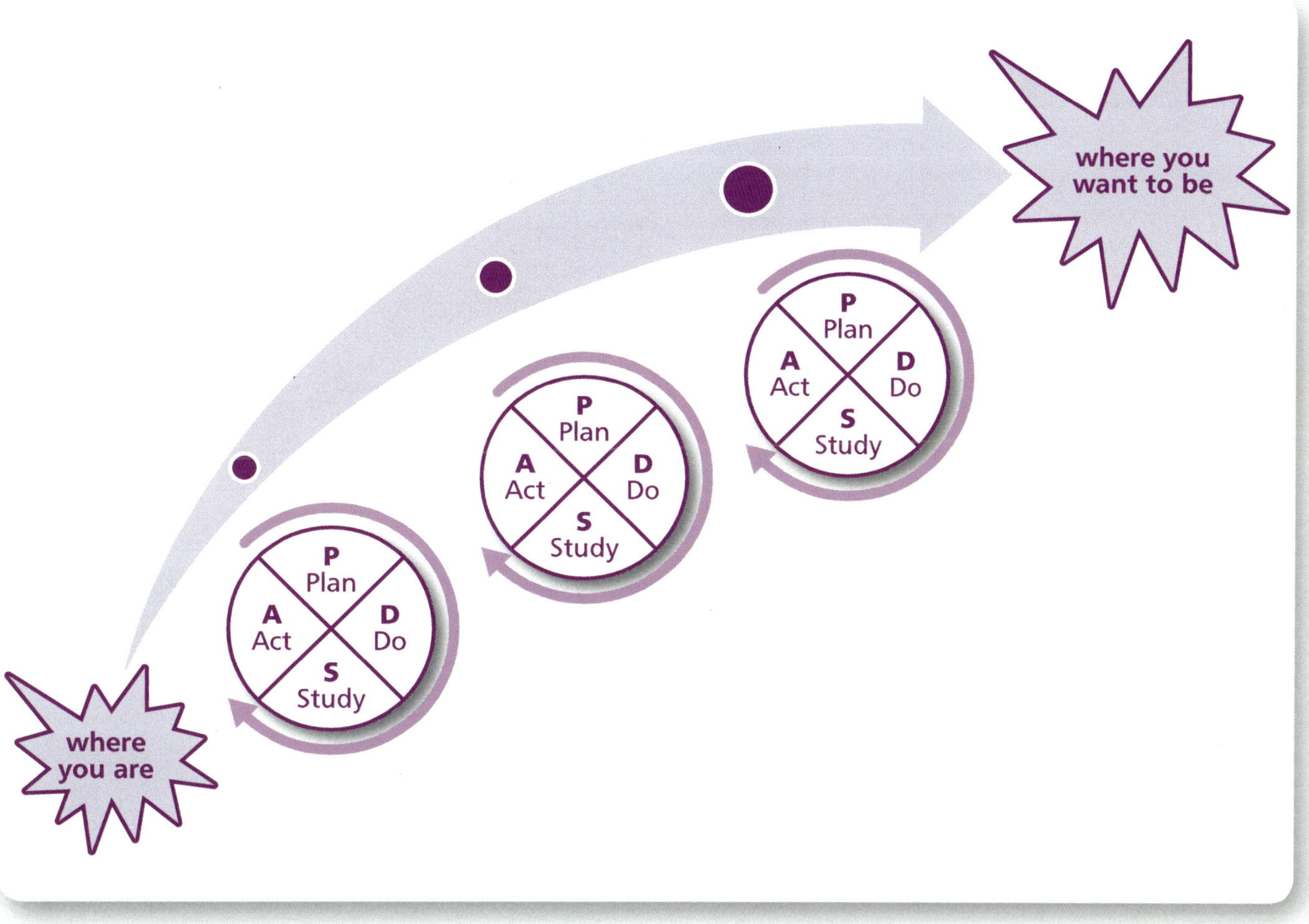
where you are
P
Plan
D
Do
S
Study
A
Act
P
Plan
D
Do
S
Study
A
Act
P
Plan
D
Do
S
Study
A
Act
where you want to be

Table 1. Categories of the *Quality* Book of Tools resourced from the Health Quality Ontario (HQO) [formerly Ontario Health Quality Council (OHQC)] and the Institute of Medicine

Quality Book of Tools	Health Quality Ontario (HQO) [formerly Ontario Health Quality Council (OHQC)]	Institute of Medicine (IOM)
Category A: Patient-Centred Practice issues include privacy and confidentiality, guiding documents and legal contracts, mandatory reporting and boundary issues. Patient issues include feedback and input, informed decision making and self-management, and the provision of educational resources.	**Patient-Centred** Health-care providers should offer services in a way that is sensitive to an individual's needs and preferences. For example, you should receive care that respects your dignity and privacy. You should be able to find care that respects your religious, cultural and language needs and your life's circumstances.	**Patient-Centred** Providing care that is respectful of and responsive to individual patient preferences, needs, and values and ensuring that patient values guide all clinical decisions.
Category B: Equitable Patients are accepted and treated in the practice without discrimination regardless of who they are and where they live, and, when required, are given extra services.	**Equitable** People should get the same quality of care regardless of who they are and where they live. For example, if you don't speak English or French it can be hard to find out about the health services you need and to get to those services. The same can be true for people who are poor or less educated, or for those who live in small or far-off communities. Extra help is sometimes needed to make sure everyone gets the care they need.	**Equitable** Providing care that does not vary in quality because of personal characteristics such as gender, ethnicity, geographic location, and socioeconomic status.
Category C: Timely and Accessible Patients obtain appointments, referrals, test results and after-hours or emergency care in a timely manner. New patients' medical records are transferred efficiently.	**Accessible** People should be able to get the right care at the right time in the right setting by the right health-care provider. For example, when a special test is needed, you should receive it when needed and without causing you extra strain and upset. If you have a chronic illness such as diabetes or asthma, you should be able to find help to manage your disease and avoid more serious problems.	**Timely** Reducing waits and sometimes harmful delays for both those who receive and those who give care.
Category D: Safe Safety issues include infection control, vaccine storage, performance of office procedures, disposal of sharps and medical waste, safe and appropriate medical equipment, drug and prescription management, medical record storage, ensuring medical records include essential information, tracking test results and incident reporting.	**Safe** People should not be harmed by an accident or mistakes when they receive care.	**Safe** Avoiding injuries to patients from the care that is intended to help them.

Quality Book of Tools	Health Quality Ontario (HQO) [formerly Ontario Health Quality Council (OHQC)]	Institute of Medicine (IOM)
Category E: Effective Clinical Practice Patients receive quality clinical care based on best-practice evidence-based guidelines and include the clinical outcomes of lifestyle and prevention, immunization, screening and surveillance, life-cycle clinical management, sexual health, family violence, chronic disease management and palliative care.	**Effective** People should receive care that works and is based on the best available scientific information. For example, your doctor (or healthcare provider) should know what the proven treatments are for your particular needs including best ways of coordinating care, preventing disease or using technology. **Focused on population health** The health system should work to prevent sickness and improve the health of the people of Ontario.	**Effective** Providing services based on scientific knowledge to all who could benefit and refraining from providing services to those not likely to benefit (avoiding underuse and overuse, respectively).
Category F: Efficient Tests and reports are managed and accessed efficiently, avoiding unnecessary duplication and time wastage.	**Efficient** The health system should continually look for ways to reduce waste, including waste of supplies, equipment, time, ideas and information. For example, to avoid the need to repeat tests or wait for reports to be sent from one doctor to another, your health information should be available to all of your doctors through a secure computer system.	**Efficient** Avoiding waste, including waste of equipment, supplies, ideas and energy.
Category G: Integrated and Continuous Indicators include integration and continuity of care, including services for patients with complex needs, integration with community care and provision of out-of-office care.	**Integrated** All parts of the health system should be organized, connected and work with one another to provide high-quality care. For example, if you need major surgery, your care should be managed so that you move smoothly from hospital to rehabilitation and into the care you need after you go home.	
Category H: Appropriate Practice Resources Indicators include human resources management, physical facilities, workplace safety and fire management, and practice improvement and planning.	**Appropriately resourced** The health system should have enough qualified providers, funding, information, equipment, supplies and facilities to look after people's health needs. For example, as people age they develop more health problems. This means there will be more need for specialized machines, doctors, nurses and others to provide good care. A high-quality health system will plan and prepare for this.	

Figure 1. Categories and Indicators

A — Patient-Centred

7 Sub-categories – 8 Indicators

A.1 Privacy and Confidentiality

- The practice team maintains the privacy of patient information in accordance with legislation

A.2 Guiding Documents and Legal Contracts

- The practice team demonstrates its commitment to respecting the needs and rights of its patients

A.3 Mandatory Reporting

- Mandatory reporting occurs in accordance with legislation

A.4 Boundary Issues

- All members of the clinical team are trained in professional standards regarding boundary issues

A.5 Encouraging Patient Feedback and Suggestions

- The practice team encourages patient feedback and suggestions
- The practice team respects patients' rights to complain

A.6 Informed Decision Making

- Patients are provided with enough information to make informed decisions about their care

A.7 Educational Resources for Patients

- The clinical team provides educational information on health

B — Equitable

1 Sub-category – 3 Indicators

B.1 Equitable Care

- New patients are accepted into the practice without discrimination
- Patients get the same quality of care regardless of who they are and where they live
- The clinical team identifies and provides additional services for patients with special needs

C — Timely and Accessible

2 Sub-categories – 6 Indicators

C.1 Timely and Accessible

- Patients can reach the practice by telephone, email and/or other electronic means
- Patients can book appropriate appointments
- Registration of new patients and transfer of medical records are timely and accessible
- Investigations and referrals occur in a timely manner

C.2 After-Hours and Emergency Care

- The clinical team provides access to 24-hour care, 7 days a week
- The practice team responds to emergencies and urgent medical conditions

D — Safe

8 Sub-categories – 11 Indicators

D.1 Infection Control

- The practice team follows infection-control guidelines

D.2 Cold Chain

- The practice team follows provincial guidelines for vaccine storage/cold chain

D.3 Office Procedures

- Procedures performed in the office conform to accepted guidelines

D.4 Disposal of Sharps and Medical Waste

- The practice team safely disposes of sharps and biomedical waste

D.5 Medical Equipment

- Medical equipment and resources are safe, appropriate, secure, available and maintained

D.6 Drugs

- Drugs available in the practice are appropriate, controlled, secure and maintained
- Prescription management

D.7 Medical Record-keeping

- Medical records are stored or filed safely and securely
- Medical records include all essential information necessary to provide quality patient care
- There is a system to track and manage patient test results and medical reports

D.8 Incident Reporting

- There is an incident reporting system to identify and address serious or potentially serious adverse events

E
Effective Clinical Practice

9 Sub-categories – 27 Indicators

E.1 Lifestyle and Prevention
- Smoking cessation
- Alcohol
- Diet and exercise

E.2 Immunization
- Baby, childhood and adolescent immunizations
- Adult immunizations

E.3 Surveillance and Screening
- Screening for colorectal cancer
- Screening for cervical cancer
- Screening for breast cancer

E.4 Life Cycle Clinical Management
- Well baby/child care
- Adolescent care
- Maternity care
- Adult care
- Frail elder care

E.5 Sexual Health
- Sexual Health

E.6 Family Violence
- Family Violence

E.7 Chronic Disease Management
- Mental health
- Diabetes mellitus
- Hypertension
- Secondary prevention in coronary heart disease (CHD)
- Stroke or transient ischemic attacks (TIAs)
- Asthma
- Chronic obstructive pulmonary disease (COPD)
- Hypothyroidism
- Epilepsy
- Cancer

E.8 Palliative Care
- Palliative care

E.9 Open Indicator
- Open Indicator

F
Efficient

1 Sub-category – 1 Indicator

F.1 Efficient Information Management
- There is a system to manage patients' tests and reports efficiently

G
Integrated & Continuous

2 Sub-categories – 3 Indicators

G.1 Continuity of Care in the Office
- The practice team provides continuity of care
- The practice team provides continuity of care to patients with complex needs (high-frequency users, regular emergency users, patients often in crisis, and patients with multiple problems)

G.2 Out-of-Office Care
- There is a policy for out-of-office care

H
Appropriate Practice Resources

4 Sub-categories – 11 Indicators

H.1 Human Resources Management
- All clinical team members of the practice are qualified and certified
- The practice team has human resources policies and procedures
- The practice members function as a team
- The practice team members balance work and home life

H.2 Physical Facilities
- The practice is physically accessible
- The practice's waiting area accommodates patients and their family members
- Examination areas ensure patient comfort and privacy

H.3 Workplace Safety and Fire Management
- The practice is committed to workplace safety
- Fire risk is minimized

H.4 Practice Improvement and Planning
- The practice team promotes continuous quality improvement (CQI)
- The practice team has a formulated practice plan for improvement and risk management

This chart illustrates the categories, sub-categories and indicators of the *Quality* Book of Tools.
There are 70 performance indicators: 43 practice management and 27 clinical indicators

SUMMARY OF CATEGORIES AND INDICATORS

Category A: Patient-Centred

Indicators in this category cover practice and patient issues: Practice issues include privacy and confidentiality, guiding documents and legal contracts, mandatory reporting and boundary issues; patient issues include feedback and input, informed decision making and self-management, and the provision of educational resources.

Category A has 7 Sub-Categories with 8 Indicators

A.1 Privacy and Confidentiality

Indicator A.1.1

The practice team maintains the privacy of patient information in accordance with legislation

Recommended steps for maintaining patient privacy include drafting a written policy, training staff, obtaining patient consent for the release of notes to third parties, and protecting personal records.

A.2 Guiding Documents and Legal Contracts

Indicator A.2.1

The practice team demonstrates its commitment to respecting the needs and rights of its patients

Team members are dedicated to comprehensive care and the rights of patients, and are knowledgeable about the practice's services, legal obligations and contractual requirements.

A.3 Mandatory Reporting

Indicator A.3.1

Mandatory reporting occurs in accordance with legislation

Clinical team members are familiar with regulatory guidelines and record reported cases.

A.4 Boundary Issues

Indicator A.4.1

All members of the clinical team are trained in professional standards regarding boundary issues

Clinical team members are familiar with the boundaries policies of their regulatory colleges; practice management knows how to recognize and disclose conflicts of interest.

A.5 Encouraging Patient Feedback and Suggestions

Indicator A.5.1

The practice team encourages patient feedback and suggestions

Patients can suggest improvements via questionnaires, committees or suggestion boxes; the practice documents patients' feedback and communicates it to team members.

Indicator A.5.2

The practice team respects patients' rights to complain

The practice has a documented complaints policy and records all complaints and their resolution.

A.6 Informed Decision Making

Indicator A.6.1

Patients are provided with enough information to make informed decisions about their care

Patients receive sufficient information and support to make informed decisions and give informed consent; appropriate forms are provided.

A.7 Educational Resources for Patients

Indicator A.7.1

The clinical team provides educational information on health promotion and prevention and disease management

Patients receive educational materials, community referrals, written and online resources and information about available public health programs.

Category B: Equitable Care

Indicators in this category cover equity issues: Patients are accepted and treated without discrimination regardless of who they are and where they live and, when required, are given extra services.

Category B has 1 Sub-Category with 3 Indicators

B.1 Equitable Care

Indicator B.1.1

New patients are accepted into the practice without discrimination

All clinical team members are aware of their professional obligations to accept new patients into the practice.

Indicator B.1.2

Patients get the same quality of care regardless of who they are and where they live

The quality of care is the same for all patients, including immigrants, refugees, the homeless and Aboriginal Peoples; quality is not influenced by patients' sexual orientation, gender, age, language or religion.

Indicator B.1.3

The clinical team identifies and provides additional services for patients with special needs

The clinical team can provide additional services as required for patients with special needs including cultural issues and language, impaired vision and hearing, and physical and cognitive disabilities.

Category C: Timely and Accessible

Indicators in this category cover issues of timeliness and accessibility: Patients receive appointments, referrals, test results and after-hours or emergency care in a timely manner, and new patients' medical records are transferred efficiently.

Category C has 2 Sub-Categories with 6 Indicators

C.1 Timely and Accessible

Indicator C.1.1
Patients can reach the practice by telephone, email and/or other electronic means
The telephone system, email and/or other electronic systems are user-friendly and facilitate easy access to the practice.

Indicator C.1.2
Patients can book appropriate appointments
Patients can book longer or shorter appointments as needed and wait-times are monitored.

Indicator C.1.3
Registration of new patients and transfer of medical records are timely and accessible
New patients are registered efficiently and their medical records are transferred to and from the practice according to CPSO guidelines.

Indicator C.1.4
Investigations and referrals occur in a timely manner
There is a system in place to monitor wait times for investigations and referrals.

C.2 After-Hours and Emergency Care

Indicator C.2.1
The clinical team provides access to 24-hour care, seven days a week
The practice ensures access to 24/7 medical care; alternative arrangements are provided if the clinical team does not provide 24-hour care.

Indicator C.2.2
The practice team responds to emergencies and urgent medical conditions
Patients are able to book urgent-care visits; the practice team is trained to recognize and respond to emergencies.

Category D: Safe

Indicators in this category cover safety issues: infection control, vaccine storage, office procedures, disposal of sharps and medical waste, safe and appropriate medical equipment, drug and prescription management, medical record storage, ensuring essential information is included in medical records, tracking test results and incident reporting.

Category D has 8 Sub-Categories with 11 Indicators

D.1 Infection Control

Indicator D.1.1 – The practice team follows infection-control guidelines

Team members follow disinfection and sterilization guidelines, store sterile instruments appropriately and practise hand hygiene.

D.2 Cold Chain

Indicator D.2.1 – The practice team follows provincial guidelines for vaccine storage/cold chain

Guidelines for effective vaccine storage include using a designated refrigerator and ensuring that vaccines are current.

D.3 Office Procedures

Indicator D.3.1 – Procedures performed in the office conform to accepted guidelines

The practice has a list of approved procedures, and clinical team members have suitable training and equipment to perform these procedures in accordance with accepted guidelines.

D.4 Disposal of Sharps & Biomedical Waste

Indicator D.4.1 – The practice team safely disposes of sharps and biomedical waste

The practice team has a system to safely dispose of sharps and contaminated materials.

D.5 Medical Equipment

Indicator D.5.1 – Medical equipment & resources are safe, appropriate, secure, available and maintained

The practice's medical equipment is safe, appropriate, available when required, and well-maintained.

D.6 Drugs

Indicator D.6.1 – Drugs available in the practice are appropriate, controlled, secure and maintained

Recommended steps for controlling drugs in the practice include authorized access, secure storage, a bi-annual audit, and dispensing records.

Indicator D.6.2 – Prescription management

Medications ordered for patients are prescribed and managed in the safest manner possible.

D.7 Medical Record-keeping

Indicator D.7.1 – Medical records are stored or filed safely and securely

Recommended steps to ensure that medical records are stored securely and retrievable only by authorized medical staff include safe storage of backup tapes or CDs, computer password protection and lockouts, and an IT strategic plan.

Indicator D.7.2

Medical records include all essential information necessary to provide quality patient care

Patient records should include cumulative patient profiles, up-to-date lists of problems and medications, telephone conversations, clinical decisions and all other necessary information about the patient and their care in accordance with best-practice guidelines, legal and local standards.

Indicator D.7.3

There is a system to track and manage patient test results and medical reports

The practice has an effective system in place for managing test results and medical reports, including follow-up of missing results and notification of patients.

D.8 Incident Reporting

Indicator D.8.1

There is an incident reporting system to identify and address serious or potentially serious adverse events

An incident reporting and management system is in place that identifies and addresses adverse events, errors, near-misses, etc.

Category E: Effective Clinical Practice

Indicators in this category recommend steps for ensuring that patients receive quality care based on best-practice evidence-based guidelines, and include the clinical outcomes of lifestyle and prevention, immunization, screening and surveillance, life-cycle clinical management, sexual health, family violence, chronic disease management and palliative care.

Category E has 9 Sub-Categories with 27 Indicators

E.1 Lifestyle and Prevention

Indicator E.1.1
Smoking cessation
The practice team uses an evidence-based approach to help patients quit smoking, and monitors their progress.

Indicator E.1.2
Alcohol
Recommended ways in which the practice can help patients with alcohol use and abuse problems include screening tools, counselling, medication and referrals to community programs.

Indicator E.1.3
Diet and exercise
Recommended ways in which the practice can help patients with diet and exercise include a regular assessment of medication, referrals to community resources, and the recording of BMI and waist circumference.

E.2 Immunization

Indicator E.2.1
Baby, childhood and adolescent immunizations
The practice team meets the provincial guidelines for baby, childhood and adolescent immunizations, including providing Public Health with regular updates and reporting adverse reactions.

Indicator E.2.2
Adult immunizations
The practice team meets the provincial guidelines for adult immunizations, including reporting adverse reactions to Health Canada.

E.3 Surveillance and Screening

Indicator E.3.1 – Screening for colorectal cancer
The practice team meets the provincial guidelines for screening, surveillance and recall for early detection of colorectal cancer.

Indicator E.3.2 – Screening for cervical cancer
The practice team meets the provincial guidelines for screening, surveillance and recall for early detection of cervical cancer.

Indicator E.3.3 – Screening for breast cancer
The practice team meets the provincial guidelines for screening, surveillance and recall for early detection of breast cancer.

E.4 Life Cycle Clinical Management

Indicator E.4.1 – Well baby/child care
The practice team meets the provincial best-practice guidelines for well baby/child care.

Indicator E.4.2 – Adolescent care
The practice team meets the best-practice guidelines for adolescent care, including sexual health care, immunizations, prescription management, and referrals to Children's Aid.

Indicator E.4.3 – Maternity care
The practice team meets the provincial best-practice guidelines for maternity care, including prenatal screenings and referrals to other care providers.

Indicator E.4.4 – Adult care
The clinical team meets the best-practice guidelines for the care of both men and women.

Indicator E.4.5 – Frail elder care
The clinical team meets the best-practice guidelines for care of the frail elderly, including identifying vulnerable older patients, assessing their cognitive ability, and monitoring medications.

E.5 Sexual Health

Indicator E.5.1 – Sexual health
The provision of sexual health care includes testing and follow-up for HIV/AIDS and STIs, and family planning.

E.6 Family Violence

Indicator E.6.1
Family violence
The clinical team routinely screens, manages and follows up on victims of family violence.

E.7 Chronic Disease Management

Indicator E.7.1
Mental health
Best-practice guidelines for the care of patients with mental health disorders include regular medication assessment and shared-care with psychiatrists and other mental health professionals.

Indicator E.7.2
Diabetes mellitus
Screening and care management for patients with diabetes includes shared-care with specialists and other health professionals and a system for regularly updating patients' records with lab results and other benchmarks.

Indicator E.7.3
Hypertension
The clinical team meets best-practice guidelines for patients with hypertension, including regular medication assessments.

Indicator E.7.4
Secondary prevention in coronary heart disease (CHD)
The clinical team meets the best-practice guidelines for patients with coronary heart disease (CHD), including regular medication assessments and an annual audit of care.

Indicator E.7.5
Stroke or transient ischemic attacks (TIAs)
Best practice-guidelines for patients with stroke or transient ischemic attacks include a system for care management, regular medication assessments and an annual audit of stroke and TIA patients' records.

Indicator E.7.6
Asthma
Best-practice guidelines for patients with asthma include a system for care management, regular medication assessments and advice on lifestyle modification.

Indicator E.7.7
Chronic obstructive pulmonary disease (COPD)
Recommended management of patients with chronic obstructive pulmonary disease includes shared-care with specialists, medication assessments and lifestyle modification advice.

Indicator E.7.8
Hypothyroidism
Recommended management of patients with hypothyroidism includes shared-care with specialists and regular medication assessments.

Indicator E.7.9
Epilepsy
Recommended management of patients with epilepsy includes shared-care with specialists, regular medication assessments and an annual audit of patients' records.

Indicator E.7.10 Cancer
Best-practice guidelines for patients with cancer include shared-care with specialists, medication assessments, and carefully maintained records of diagnosis, ongoing treatment and after-care.

E.8 Palliative Care

Indicator E.8.1
Palliative care
Recommended management of palliative care patients includes a system of referrals and shared-care and regular medication assessments.

E.9 Open Indicator

Indicator E.9.1
Open indicator
This generic indicator allows the practice team to adapt and apply the framework developed for each indicator to other clinical problems or issues identified as important and relevant to the practice.

Category F: Efficient

The indicator in this category ensures tests and reports are managed efficiently to avoid unnecessary duplication and time wastage.

Category F has 1 Sub-Category with 1 Indicator

F.1 Efficient Information Management

Indicator F.1.1
There is a system to manage patients' tests and reports efficiently
The practice has established procedures to manage patients' test results and reports, avoid duplication of tests and manage appointments efficiently.

Category G: Integrated and Continuous

Indicators in this category ensure integration and continuity of care, including services for patients with complex needs, integration with community care and the provision of out-of-office care.

Category G has 2 Sub-Categories with 3 Indicators

G.1 Continuity of Care in the Office

Indicator G.1.1

The practice team provides continuity of care

The practice team provides continuous, comprehensive and coordinated medical care, including links with hospital-based services, specialists and community-based agencies. Patients have the opportunity to develop an ongoing relationship with the practice team members.

Indicator G.1.2

The practice team provides continuity of care to patients with complex needs (high-frequency users, regular emergency users, patients often in crisis, and patients with multiple problems)

A system of alerts and management of after-hours care ensures continuous, comprehensive and coordinated medical care for patients with complex needs.

G.2 Out-of-Office Care

Indicator G.2.1

There is a policy for out-of-office care

The practice has a system to ensure patients can be treated at home, in hospital, in rehabilitation and other settings.

Category H: Appropriate Practice Resources

Indicators in this category cover human resources management, physical facilities, workplace safety and fire management, and practice improvement and planning.

Category H has 4 Sub-Categories with 11 Indicators

H.1 Human Resources Management

Indicator H.1.1
All clinical team members of the practice are qualified and certified
Clinical team members are qualified and certified, and maintain updated licences, credentials and privileges.

Indicator H.1.2
The practice has human resources policies and procedures
The practice team has human resources policies and procedures, including documented workplace policies and signed employment contracts for each practice member.

Indicator H.1.3
The practice members function as a team
The practice members function as a team; regular practice meetings are provided and recorded.

Indicator H.1.4
The practice team members balance work and home life
The practice team members balance work and home life; part-time and flexible work hours are supported, and parental needs incorporated into planning.

H.2 Physical Facilities

Indicator H.2.1
The practice is physically accessible
The practice is physically accessible to most patients, including those with mobility problems.

Indicator H.2.2
The practice's waiting area accommodates patients and their family members
Recommendations for the waiting area include four seats per FTE doctor, and room to accommodate guide dogs and mobility scooters.

Indicator H.2.3
Examination areas ensure patients' comfort and privacy
Examination room is comfortable and private; conversations cannot be overheard.

H.3 Workplace Safety and Fire Management

Indicator H.3.1
The practice is committed to meet workplace safety
Workplace Safety and Insurance Board (WSIB) and Occupational Health and Safety Act (OHSA) requirements.

Indicator H.3.2
Fire risk is minimized
Recommendations for fire safety include an approved evacuation plan and appropriate fire-protection equipment.

H.4 Practice Improvement and Planning

Indicator H.4.1
The practice team promotes continuous quality improvement (CQI)
There is a designated person responsible for ensuring the practice team promotes a culture of continuous quality improvement (CQI).

Indicator H.4.2
The practice team has a formulated practice plan for improvement and risk management
The practice team undergoes regular purposeful planning for improvement and risk management, including disaster planning.

Audit

An audit is an official, systematic examination of the record of any aspect of patient care. A clinical audit is conducted by a family practice to identify opportunities for improving the medical care provided to patients and to provide a mechanism for realizing those improvements. In the *Quality* Book of Tools, we recommend regular audits – annual, biannual (twice a year) and biennial (every two years), for instance – as a means of assessing whether the criterion has been met. Then a plan must be devised to improve the audit results.

Categories

There are eight categories:
Category A – Patient-Centred
Category B – Equitable
Category C – Timely and Accessible
Category D – Safe
Category E – Effective Clinical Practice
Category F – Efficient
Category G – Integrated and Continuous
Category H – Appropriate Practice Resources

Community Care Access Centres

Community Care Access Centres (CCACs) provide a simplified service-access point. They are responsible for determining patient eligibility for services; buying (on behalf of consumers) the highest-quality, best-priced visiting professional and homemaker services provided at home and in publicly funded schools; determining eligibility for, and authorizing all admissions to long-term care facilities (nursing homes and homes for the aged); planning services and case management for each client; and providing information on and referral to all other long-term care services (including volunteer-based community services).

Ontario Association of Community Care Access Centres. Main Page [Internet]. [cited 2010 Jul 21].
Available from: **http://oaccac.on.ca/**

Consumer

Any patient who actually or potentially receives primary care

Continuous Quality Improvement (CQI)

CQI is the process of collecting data about a particular practice or service to benchmark performance, tracking and validating indicators that affect outcomes, and recognizing problems in processes of care and practice management. The culture of CQI is of never-ending improvement of the whole system as part of normal daily activity, continually striving to act according to the best available knowledge.

Criteria

Criteria are the elements of care that can be counted or measured in order to assess the Indicator. They are discrete, definable, measurable and explicit. A criterion should be so clearly defined that we can say definitively whether it is present or not. These criteria were adopted from the NZ Aiming for Excellence [7] and refined by the authors in the development of the *Quality* Book of Tools.

There are three types of Criteria:

- ⚖ **Legal and Safety** – required by law*
- ★ **Essential** – required to demonstrate best practice
- ❃ **Desirable** – required to demonstrate additional quality

*(*Assumptions about ⚖ indicators are based on the nature of these indicators and the regulations that qualify them)*

Drugs

In this book we have chosen to use the sub-category heading "Drugs" to encompass all prescription and non-prescription medications (over-the-counter, herbal and street drugs).

Family Health Group (FHG)

An enhanced fee-for-service model offered to groups of three or more physicians to provide comprehensive primary care to their enrolled/assigned patients 24/7 through a combination of regular office hours, after-hours services and access to the Telephone Health Advisory Service (THAS).

Family Health Network (FHN)

A blended capitation payment model for groups of three or more physicians offering patients care 24/7 through a combination of regular physician office hours, after-hours services and access to a registered nurse toll-free through THAS.

Family Health Organization (FHO)

Similar to the FHN; however, including a different base rate payment associated with a larger basket of core services.

Family Health Team (FHT)

A Family Health Team (FHT) brings together various interdisciplinary health-care providers to coordinate enhanced quality of care for the patient. FHTs consist of physicians working with other providers such as:

- Nurses, nurse practitioners
- Dietitians
- Mental health workers
- Social workers
- Pharmacists
- Educators and others
- Specialists

FHTs may choose from three governance structures:

- Community-led groups
- Provider-led groups
- Mix of provider groups and community groups

Ministry of Health & Long-Term Care (Ontario). Family Health Teams [Internet]. 2002
[updated 2014 Jul 08; cited 2014 Jul 09].
Available from:
www.health.gov.on.ca/en/pro/programs/fht/

Family Practice

A family practice consists of the physical space and the people (health-care providers and staff) who provide family medicine/primary care services in one location. The interdisciplinary primary care professionals who work in a family practice include family physicians, nurse practitioners, family practice nurses, registered practical nurses, social workers, dietitians, pharmacists, specialists, educators and others. Staff members include receptionists, practice managers and administrative support.

Fee-For-Service

The method of billing for health services whereby a physician or other practitioner charges the Ontario Health Insurance Plan (OHIP) or the patient for each patient encounter or service rendered.

Further Information

Each indicator has a section that provides links to the most useful Canadian or international sites with further information to guide the practice. These have been reviewed and are up to date as of the publication of this book. The most frequently cited references and sites include: CPSO, CMPA, OMA, OCFP, QIIP, *Canadian Family Physician* and *American Family Physician*, and The Cochrane Library.

Guidelines

Guidelines are "systematically developed statements to assist practitioners and patient decisions about appropriate health care for specific circumstances."[5] Guidelines are a summary of the recommendations based on the evidence for best practice in clinical settings.

Indicators

Clinical indicators assess particular health structures, processes and outcomes. They can be rate- or mean-based, providing a quantitative basis for quality improvement, or sentinel, identifying incidents of care that trigger further investigation. They can assess aspects of the structure, process, or outcome of health care. Further, indicators can be generic measures that are relevant for most patients or disease-specific, expressing the quality of care for patients with specific diagnoses.[6] In the *Quality* Book of Tools there are two types of indicators: practice management and clinical. They identify elements of practice performance for which there is evidence or consensus that can be used to assess and produce a change in the quality of care provided. Indicators define the practice issue or disease to be assessed. The indicators are organized into eight categories and 34 sub-categories.

Outcomes

Outcomes are all possible demonstrable results that stem from causal factors or activities.

Patient

A patient is someone who identifies the practice (the family doctor, nurse practitioner and other members of the clinical team) as their primary care provider. The patient may be in a fee-for-service practice or "rostered/ enrolled" in a FHG, FHN, FHO, FHT. For some clinical providers it is more appropriate to refer to patients as "clients."

Patient Satisfaction Questionnaire/Survey

This questionnaire is used to assess patient satisfaction with different aspects of their health care. In the tool, we recommend that patient satisfaction surveys be used to obtain feedback and suggestions on the quality of services provided by the practice. We recommend regular surveys (annual, bi-annual, or as needed when making changes, etc.).

Plan, Do, Study, Act (PDSA)

A number of models and cycles can be used in an ongoing way in order to apply CQI. One of the most commonly used approaches that has been successful in family practice settings is the Plan-Do-Study-Act (PDSA) cycle. The PDSA cycle enables change by developing a plan to test the change (Plan), carrying out the test (Do), observing and learning from the consequences (Study), and determining what modifications should be made to the test (Act).

Institute for Healthcare Improvement. Plan-Do-Study-Act (PDSA) Worksheet (IHI Tool) [Internet]. [cited 2010 Jul 21]. Available from: **www.ihi.org/IHI/Topics/Improvement/ImprovementMethods/Tools/Plan-Do-Study-Act+(PDSA)+Worksheet.htm**

Sub-Category

The *Quality* Book of Tools has Sub-Categories which further define the categories. The sub-categories group similar indicators.

Team

A team is a group of people with different skills and different tasks who work together on a common project, service, or goal, with a meshing of functions and mutual support. In the tool, we refer to teams in different ways: "the clinical team"; "the practice" or "the practice team."

- The clinical team refers to all the clinical health professionals providing care to patients in the practice.
- The practice team refers to all the clinical health professionals and staff members in the practice. "The practice team can describe" means that all members of the practice are familiar with and can describe a policy or process in a criterion.

The Practice

The practice refers to the family practice building, the practice team and all activities undertaken as part of the family practice.

The Practice Management

The practice management refers to the leadership responsible for maintaining quality in the practice. The practice management is responsible for producing written policies, reports, etc.

Urgent Care

Urgent care is medical care for a condition which is not an emergency but is severe or painful enough to require treatment or evaluation within a reasonable period of time, in order to avoid serious deterioration in the patient's condition or health.

AAFP	American Academy of Family Physicians
ACE	Angiotensin-Converting-Enzyme
AIDS	Acquired Immune Deficiency Syndrome
BC	British Columbia
BCLS	Basic Cardiac Life Support
BMI	Body Mass Index
BMA	British Medical Association
BMJ	British Medical Journal
BP	Blood Pressure
CCAC	Community Care Access Centre
CCO	Cancer Care Ontario
CD	Compact Disc
CDO	College of Dietitians of Ontario
CFP	Canadian Family Physician
CFPC	College of Family Physicians of Canada
CFSA	Child and Family Services Act
CHD	Coronary Heart Disease
CMA	Canadian Medical Association
CMAJ	Canadian Medical Association Journal
CMPA	Canadian Medical Protective Association
CNA	Canadian Nurses Association
CNO	College of Nurses of Ontario
CNPS	Canadian Nurses Protective Society
CO	Carbon Monoxide
COPD	Chronic Obstructive Pulmonary Disease
CPD	Continuous Professional Development
CPhA	Canadian Pharmacists Association
CPP	Cumulative Patient Profile
CPR	Cardio Pulmonary Resuscitation
CPSO	College of Physicians & Surgeons of Ontario
CQI	Continuous Quality Improvement
CT	Computed Tomography
DNR	Do Not Resuscitate
EBM	(McMaster) Espresso Book Maker
EMR	Electronic Medical Records
EPA	European Practice Assessment
ESAS	Edmonton Symptom Assessment System
FHG	Family Health Group
FHN	Family Health Network
FHO	Family Health Organization
FHT	Family Health Team
FOBT	Fecal Occult Blood Test
FTE	Full-Time Equivalent
HbA1c	Haemoglobin A1c
HDL	High Density Lipoprotein
HIPA	Health Information Protection Act
HIV	Human Immunodeficiency Virus
HPV	Human Papilloma Virus
HQO	Health Quality Ontario
ICSI	Institute for Clinical Systems Improvement
IHI	Institute for Healthcare Improvement
INR	International Normalized Ratio
IOM	Institute of Medicine
IUD	Intra-Uterine Device
IT	Information Technology
JAMA	Journal of the American Medical Association
LDL	Low Density Lipoprotein
MOHLTC	Ministry of Health & Long-Term Care
MRI	Magnetic Resonance Imaging
NP	Nurse Practitioner
OCFP	Ontario College of Family Physicians
OCP	Ontario College of Pharmacists
OFM	Office of the Fire Marshall
OHIP	Ontario Health Insurance Plan
OHSA	Occupational Health and Safety Act
OMA	Ontario Medical Association
OCSWSSW	Ontario College of Social Workers and Social Service Workers
PCN	Primary Care Network
PDSA	Plan-Do-Study-Act
PHAC	Public Health Agency of Canada
QA	Quality Assurance
QCIPA	Quality of Care Information Protection Act
QIIP	Quality Improvement & Innovation Partnership
RACGP	Royal Australian College of General Practitioners
RN	Registered Nurse
RNZCGP	Royal New Zealand College of General Practitioners
SARS	Severe Acute Respiratory Syndrome
SOGC	Society of Obstetricians and Gynaecologists of Canada
THAS	Telephone Health Advisory Service
TIA	Transient Ischemic Attack
TB	Tuberculosis
USA	United States of America
UK	United Kingdom
WHMIS	Workplace Hazardous Materials Information System
WHO	World Health Organization
WSIB	Workplace Safety and Insurance Board

REFERENCES

1. Institute of Medicine. Crossing the Quality Chasm: Establishing Aims for the 21st century Health Care System [monograph online]. Washington (DC): National Academy Press; 2001 [cited 2010 Jul 21]. Available from: **www.nap.edu/openbook.php?isbn=0309072808**.
2. Health Quality Ontario: Quality Monitor 2012 Report on Ontario's Health System [Internet]. 2012 [cited 2014 Jul 09]. Available from: **www.hqontario.ca/portals/0/Documents/pr/qmonitor-full-report-2012-en.pdf**
3. Berwick DM. A Primer on Leading the Improvement of Systems. BMJ. 1996;312:619-622.
4. Institute for Healthcare Improvement. The Breakthrough Series: IHI's Collaborative Model for Achieving Breakthrough Improvement. Diabetes Spectrum. 2004;17(2):97-101.
5. Field MJ, Lohr KN, editor. Clinical Practice Guidelines: Directions for a New Program. Institute of Medicine. Washington (DC): National Academy Press, 1990.
6. Mainz J. Defining and classifying clinical indicators for quality improvement. International Journal for Quality in Health Care. 2003;15:523-530.
7. Royal New Zealand College of General Practitioners. Aiming for Excellence – An Assessment Tool for New Zealand General Practice. 3rd ed [monograph online]. New Zealand: Royal New Zealand College of General Practitioners (RNZCGP); 2009 [cited 2010 Jul 21]. Available from: **www.rnzcgp.org.nz/assets/documents/CORNERSTONE/Aiming-for-Excellence-2009-including-record-review.pdf**

CATEGORY A: PATIENT-CENTRED

Indicators in this category cover practice and patient issues: Practice issues include privacy and confidentiality, guiding documents and legal contracts, mandatory reporting and boundary issues; patient issues include feedback and input, informed decision making and self-management, and the provision of educational resources.

The Institute of Medicine defines patient-centred as: "Providing care that is respectful of and responsive to individual patient preferences, needs, and values and ensuring that patient values guide all clinical decisions."

The Ontario Health Quality Council says: "Health-care providers should offer services in a way that is sensitive to an individual's needs and preferences."

Category A has 7 Sub-Categories with 8 Indicators

A.1 Privacy and Confidentiality

Indicator A.1.1

The practice team maintains the privacy of patient information in accordance with legislation

Recommended steps for maintaining patient privacy include drafting a written policy, training staff, obtaining patient consent for the release of notes to third parties, and protecting personal records.

A.2 Guiding Documents and Legal Contracts

Indicator A.2.1

The practice team demonstrates its commitment to respecting the needs and rights of its patients

Team members are dedicated to comprehensive care and the rights of patients, and are knowledgeable about the practice's services, legal obligations and contractual requirements.

A.3 Mandatory Reporting

Indicator A.3.1 – Mandatory reporting occurs in accordance with legislation

Clinical team members are familiar with regulatory guidelines and record reported cases.

A.4 Boundary Issues

Indicator A.4.1

All members of the clinical team are trained in professional standards regarding boundary issues

Clinical team members are familiar with their regulatory colleges' boundaries policies; management knows how to recognize and disclose conflicts of interest.

A.5 Encouraging Patient Feedback and Suggestions

Indicator A.5.1

The practice team encourages patient feedback and suggestions

Patients can suggest improvements via questionnaires, committees or suggestion boxes; the practice documents patients' feedback and communicates it to team members.

Indicator A.5.2

The practice team respects patients' rights to complain

The practice has a documented complaints policy and records all complaints and their resolution.

A.6 Informed Decision Making

Indicator A.6.1

Patients are provided with enough information to make informed decisions about their care

Patients receive sufficient information and support to make informed decisions and give informed consent; appropriate forms are provided.

A.7 Educational Resources for Patients

Indicator A.7.1

The clinical team provides educational information on health promotion and prevention and disease management

Patients receive educational materials, community referrals, written and online resources and information about available public health programs.

Sub-Category A.1 Privacy and Confidentiality

Indicator A.1.1 The practice team maintains the privacy of patient information in accordance with legislation

Criteria

- **A.1.1.1** ⚖ The practice team has been trained to maintain the privacy of patient information in accordance with legislation
- **A.1.1.2** ⚖ There is a designated contact person responsible for monitoring privacy issues
- **A.1.1.3** ⚖ The practice has a written privacy policy
- **A.1.1.4** ⚖ Patient consent is obtained and recorded before personal information and notes are released to another party
- **A.1.1.5** ⚖ The practice team takes reasonable steps to ensure records are protected
- **A.1.1.6** ⚖ The practice team has established and maintains appropriate privacy and confidentiality information and informs its patients about these practices
- **A.1.1.7** ⚖ The practice team collects and stores patients' personal information in accordance with legislation
- **A.1.1.8** ⚖ The practice team takes reasonable steps to protect personal health information that is released to others

Sub-Category A.1 Privacy and Confidentiality

Indicator A.1.1
The practice team maintains the privacy of patient information in accordance with legislation

Recommended steps for maintaining patient privacy include drafting a written policy, training staff, obtaining patient consent for the release of notes to third parties, and protecting personal records.

Criteria:

A.1.1.1 ⚖ The practice team has been trained to maintain the privacy of patient information in accordance with legislation

Interpretation

- The practice management can produce:
  - A record of training for all members of the practice
  - A record of signed confidentiality forms

A.1.1.2 ⚖ There is a designated contact person responsible for monitoring privacy issues

Interpretation

- Management and staff can identify the designated contact person

A.1.1.3 ⚖ The practice team has a written privacy policy

Interpretation

- The practice management can produce a written policy that is available to all patients and includes:
  - How the practice ensures privacy of information
  - The name of the designated contact person
  - The procedure to access, correct, inquire and complain
- The practice management can produce evidence of procedures to:
  - Identify when a disclosure of personal health information goes beyond what is described in the written statement
  - Notify affected patients about a request for disclosure
  - Keep notes of a disclosure in, or linked to, the patient's personal health record
  - Retain and dispose of private information

A.1.1.4 ⚖ Patient consent is obtained and recorded for the disclosure of personal information and the release of notes to another party

Interpretation

- The practice management can provide the results of a random chart audit that demonstrates a consent form was completed and the process recorded in the chart

Sub-Category A.1 Privacy and Confidentiality

Indicator A.1.1
The practice team maintains the privacy of patient information in accordance with legislation *(continued)*

A.1.1.5 ⚖ The practice team takes reasonable steps to ensure records are protected

Interpretation

- The practice management can describe the system to protect records against theft, loss and unauthorized access, copying, modification, use, disclosure, retention and disposal
- The practice management can produce the results of a twice-yearly audit to ensure that patient records are protected

A.1.1.6 ⚖ The practice team has established and maintains appropriate privacy and confidentiality information and informs its patients about these practices

Interpretation

- The practice posts its policy for establishing and maintaining appropriate privacy and confidentiality of information

A.1.1.7 ⚖ The practice team collects and stores patients' personal information in accordance with legislation

Interpretation

- The practice management can produce a list that defines each health-care professional's and staff member's level of access to patients' health information
- Management can describe how health information is collected and stored to other individuals or agencies requesting information (including restriction, duplication, limitations, etc.)
- Management can produce the results of an annual audit on release and collection practices

A.1.1.8 ⚖ The practice team takes reasonable steps to protect personal health information that is released to others

Interpretation

- Reasonable steps are taken to protect health information released to others
- Office staff ensures that messages left with third parties or on answering machines do not contain patients' personal health information

Sub-Category A.1 Privacy and Confidentiality

Indicator A.1.1
The practice team maintains the privacy of patient information in accordance with legislation *(continued)*

Further Information (see up to date links at **http://quality.resources.machealth.ca**)

Ministry of Health & Long-Term Care (Ontario). Personal Health Information Protection Act, 2004 [Internet]. 2004 [updated 2012 Jun 25; cited 2014 Jul 09].
Available from: **www.health.gov.on.ca/en/common/legislation/priv_legislation/**

College of Physicians & Surgeons of Ontario. Medical Records [Internet]. 2006 Mar/Apr [cited 2010 Jul 21].
Available from: **www.cpso.on.ca/policies/policies/default.aspx?id=1686**

College of Physicians and Surgeons of Ontario. Developments in Medical Record Keeping. Practice Partner [Internet]. 2009 Jul [updated 2012 May, cited 2014 Jul 09].;32-33.
Available from: **www.cpso.on.ca/CPSO/media/uploadedfiles/policies/policies/policyitems/medical_records.pdf?ext=.pdf**

College of Physicians and Surgeons of Ontario. Confidentiality of Personal Health Information [Internet]. 2006 Mar/Apr [cited 2014 Jul 09].
Available from: **www.cpso.on.ca/uploadedFiles/policies/policies/policyitems/Confidentiality.pdf**

College of Dietitians of Ontario. Practice Standards & Resources [Internet]. [updated 2010 July 14; cited 2010 Jul 21].
Available from: **www.cdo.on.ca/en/resources/practice.asp#record**

College of Nurses of Ontario. Privacy, confidentiality and your nursing practice [Internet]. 2006 Feb 17 [cited 2010 Jul 21].
Available from: **www.cno.org/Global/docs/prac/41069_privacy.pdf**

Canadian Pharmacists Association. Pharmacist's Personal Information Privacy Code [Internet]. 2004 [cited 2010 Jul 21].
Available from: **www.pharmacists.ca/cpha-ca/assets/File/PrivacyCode-2005_ENG.pdf**

Ontario College of Social Workers and Social Service Workers. Code of Ethics and Standards of Practice Handbook. 2nd ed. Ontario College of Social Workers and Social Service Workers; 2008. Principle V: Confidentiality; p.23-27. [cited 2015 May 19].
Available from: **http://ocswssw.org/wp-content/uploads/2015/01/Code-of-Ethics-Standards-of-Practice.pdf**

Canadian Medical Association. CMA Policy: Physician Guidelines for Online Communication with Patients. [Internet]. 2005 [cited 2014 Aug 26]. Available from: **https://www.cma.ca/Assets/assets-library/document/en/advocacy/CMA_online_comms_PD05-03-e.pdf#search=tools%20to%20protect%20patient%20information**

Sub-Category A.2 Guiding Documents and Legal Contracts

Indicator A.2.1 The practice team demonstrates its commitment to respecting the needs and rights of its patients

Criteria

- **A.2.1.1** ★ The practice team can describe how it provides services to patients
- **A.2.1.2** ⚖ The practice team respects the rights of patients
- **A.2.1.3** ⚖ The clinical team is familiar with its provincial contractual requirements

Further Information (see up to date links at **http://quality.resources.machealth.ca**)

Canadian Medical Association. Code of Ethics [Internet]. [updated 2004; cited 2014 Jul 09]. Available from: **https://www.cma.ca/Assets/assets-library/document/en/about-us/PD04-06-e.pdf**

Canadian Nurses Association. Code of Ethics for Registered Nurses – 2008 Centennial Edition [Internet]. [cited 2014 Jul 09]. Available from: **www.cna-aiic.ca/~/media/cna/files/en/codeofethics.pdf**

Ministry of Health & Long-Term Care (Ontario). Ontario Health Insurance Plan – Questions and Answers [Internet]. 2009 Apr [updated 2009 Dec 16; cited 2010 Jul 21]. Available from: **www.health.gov.on.ca/en/public/programs/ohip/ohipfaq_mn.aspx**

College of Physicians & Surgeons of Ontario. A Practical Guide for Safe and Effective Office-Based Practices [Internet]. 2012 May [cited 2014 Jul 09]. Available from: **www.cpso.on.ca/uploadedFiles/policies/guidelines/office/Safe-Practices.pdf**

Ministry of Health & Long-Term Care (Ontario). Family Health Teams – Advancing Primary Health Care: Guide to Patient Enrolment [Internet]. 2005 Jul 4 [cited 2014 Jul 09]. Available from: **www.health.gov.on.ca/en/pro/programs/fht/docs/fht_enrolment.pdf**

Sub-Category A.2 Guiding Documents and Legal Contracts

Indicator A.2.1
The practice team demonstrates its commitment to respecting the needs and rights of its patients

Team members are dedicated to comprehensive care and the rights of patients, and are knowledgeable about the practice's services, legal obligations and contractual requirements.

Criteria:

A.2.1.1 ★ The practice team can describe how it provides services to patients

Interpretation

- The practice management can produce:
  - Written information regarding service hours, after-hours service, types of service, etc., available for patients (and routinely gives this to new patients)
  - Information about practice services, on request, in languages other than English or other formats
  - Procedures for initiating and dissolving the provider relationship
- Practice information is displayed where it can be read by patients
- Information about practice services is regularly reviewed and updated
- The practice has clearly posted guidelines and policies about payment for insured and uninsured services

A.2.1.2 ⚖ The practice team respects the rights of patients

Interpretation

- The practice respects and explains the patient's right to have a third party present during an examination or consultation
- The practice ensures that when a patient is accompanied to the practice by a third party, the patient consents to the presence of that person in an examination or consultation
- The practice management provides:
  - Privacy to undress and appropriate covering for patients during physical examinations
  - Female staff who are available to assist with examinations or consultations
- A clinic room is furnished to accommodate third parties

A.2.1.3 ⚖ The clinical team is familiar with its provincial contractual requirements

Interpretation

- The practice management can describe the provincial "model of family practice" contract within which it works, and how the practice team communicates its contractual obligations to patients. Patients should know whether they are or have agreed to be rostered and their obligations. These models include Fee-For-Service, Health Service Organization, Family Health Team, Primary Care Network, Family Health Network, Family Health Organization, Family Health Group, Community Health Centre, Community Service Contract and Northern Group Funding Plan (see Glossary).

Sub-Category A.3 Mandatory Reporting

Indicator A.3.1 Mandatory reporting occurs in accordance with legislation

Criteria A.3.1.1 ⚖ The clinical team is trained in mandatory reporting

Sub-Category A.3 Mandatory Reporting

Indicator A.3.1
Mandatory reporting occurs in accordance with legislation

Clinical team members are familiar with regulatory guidelines and record reported cases.

Criteria:

A.3.1.1 ⚖ The clinical team is trained in mandatory reporting

Interpretation

- The practice management can produce:
  - A record that the clinical team members have read their regulatory college guidelines on mandatory reporting
  - A record of the cases that have been reported

Further Information (see up to date links at **http://quality.resources.machealth.ca**)

College of Physicians & Surgeons of Ontario. Mandatory Reporting [Internet]. 2006 Jan/Feb [cited 2010 Jul 21]. Available from: **www.cpso.on.ca/uploadedFiles/policies/policies/policyitems/mandatoryreporting.pdf**

Ontario College of Social Workers and Social Service Workers. Mandatory Reports [Internet]. [cited 2010 Jul 21]. Available from: **www.ocswssw.org/employers/employers_mandatoryreporting/**

Sub-Category A.4 Boundary Issues

Indicator A.4.1 All members of the clinical team are trained in professional standards regarding boundary issues

Criteria

A.4.1.1 ★ The clinical team is familiar with boundary issues inherent in the patient-provider relationship

A.4.1.2 ★ The best interest of the patient is the foundation of patient care. This interest must not conflict with the financial or other interests of the clinical team members

Sub-Category A.4 Boundary Issues

Indicator A.4.1
All members of the clinical team are trained in professional standards regarding boundary issues

Clinical team members are familiar with the boundaries policies of their regulatory colleges; practice management knows how to recognize and disclose conflicts of interest.

Criteria:

A.4.1.1 ★ The clinical team is familiar with boundary issues inherent in the patient-provider relationship

Interpretation

- There is a record that practice members have read their regulatory college's boundaries policy
- The clinical team respects boundaries associated with limiting treatment of themselves or family members (CMA Code of Ethics)

A.4.1.2 ★ The best interest of the patient is the foundation of patient care. This interest must not conflict with the financial or other interests of the clinical team members

Interpretation

- The practice management can describe how
  - Conflicts of interest (CMA Code of Ethics) are recognized and disclosed
  - Any financial conflict (research, profit, pharmaceutical industry, formula industry) is recognized and disclosed

Further Information (see up to date links at **http://quality.resources.machealth.ca**)

College of Physicians & Surgeons of Ontario. Maintaining Appropriate Boundaries and Preventing Sexual Abuse [Internet]. 2008 Dec [cited 2014 Jul 09]. Available from: **www.cpso.on.ca/CPSO/media/uploadedfiles/policies/policies/policyitems/sexual_abuse_boundaries.pdf?ext=.pdf**

College of Physicians & Surgeons of Ontario. Maintaining Boundaries with Patients. Members' Dialogue [Internet]. 2004 Sept/Oct [cited 2014 Jul 09].;7-15. Available from: **www.cpso.on.ca/CPSO/media/images/Maintaining-Boundaries.pdf**

Canadian Medical Association. Code of Ethics [Internet]. [updated 2004; cited 2010 Jul 21]. Available from: **https://www.cma.ca/Assets/assets-library/document/en/about-us/PD04-06-e.pdf**

College of Physicians & Surgeons of Ontario. Treating Self and Family Members [Internet]. 2007Feb [cited 2010 Jul 21]. Available from: **www.cpso.on.ca/uploadedFiles/policies/policies/policyitems/treating_self.pdf**

College of Nurses of Ontario. The Standards of Care [Internet]. [cited 2014 Jul 09]. Available from: **www.cno.org/learn-about-standards-guidelines/educational-tools/learning-modules/therapeutic-nurse-client-relationship/maintaining-boundaries/**

World Health Organization. International Code on Marketing of Breastmilk Substitutes [Internet]. 1981 [cited 2010 Jul 21]. Available from: **www.who.int/nutrition/publications/code_english.pdf**

Sub-Category A.5 Encouraging Patient Feedback and Suggestions

Indicator A.5.1 The practice team encourages patient feedback and suggestions

Criteria

A.5.1.1 ❋ The practice team encourages patient feedback and suggestions

A.5.1.2 ❋ The practice team has carried out a patient-satisfaction questionnaire within the past year

A.5.1.3 ❋ Changes and improvements based on feedback and suggestions are incorporated in the practice's quality-improvement process

Sub-Category A.5 Encouraging Patient Feedback and Suggestions

Indicator A.5.1
The practice team encourages patient feedback and suggestions

Patients can suggest improvements via questionnaires, committees or suggestion boxes; the practice documents patients' feedback and communicates it to team members.

Criteria:

A.5.1.1 ❋ **The practice team encourages patient feedback and suggestions**

Interpretation

- There is a mechanism in place for patients to provide feedback and suggestions, e.g., suggestion boxes, patient participation on committees, surveys, etc.

A.5.1.2 ❋ **The practice team carries out an annual patient-satisfaction questionnaire**

Interpretation

- The practice management can produce the results of a patient-satisfaction questionnaire undertaken in the past year

A.5.1.3 ❋ **Changes and improvements based on feedback and suggestions are incorporated in the practice's quality-improvement process**

Interpretation

- The practice management can describe how:
  - Patient feedback is communicated to the practice team
  - The practice management documents all suggestions, feedback, communications, and system improvement changes

Further Information (see up to date links at **http://quality.resources.machealth.ca**)

Salisbury C, Burgess A, Lattimer V, Heaney D, Walker J, Turnbull J, Smith H. Developing a standard short questionnaire for the assessment of patient satisfaction with out-of-hours primary care. Family Practice [Internet]. 2005 [cited 2010 Jul 21];22(5):560-569.
Available from: **http://fampra.oxfordjournals.org/cgi/content/full/22/5/560** DOI:10.1093/fampra/cmi050

Ipsos MORI. The GP Patient Survey [Internet]. [cited 2010 Jul 21]. Available from: **www.gp-patient.co.uk**

Client Focused Evaluation Programme. Patient-centred Surveys - Helping People Make a Difference [Internet]. [cited 2014 Jul 09]. Available from: **www.cfepsurveys.com.au/default.aspx**

College of Physicians & Surgeons of Alberta. Physicians Achievement Review Report [Internet]. 2005 [cited 2014 Jul 09]. Available from: **http://par-program.org/par/wp-content/uploads/2014/06/Sample-GP-Report-2013.pdf**

Grogan S, Conner M, Norman P, Willits D, Porter I. Validation of a questionnaire measuring patient satisfaction with general practitioner services. Qual Health Care [Internet]. 2000 [cited 2010 Jul 21];9:210-215.
Available from: **http://qhc.bmjjournals.com/cgi/content/full/9/4/210** DOI:10.1136/qhc.9.4.210

Sub-Category A.5 Encouraging Patient Feedback and Suggestions

Indicator A.5.2 The practice team respects patients' rights to complain

Criteria

A.5.2.1 ★ The practice team has a documented complaints policy

A. 5.2.2 ★ The practice team has a designated complaints officer

A. 5.2.3 ❄ Complaints and their resolutions are incorporated in the practice quality improvement process

Sub-Category A.5 Encouraging Patient Feedback and Suggestions

Indicator A.5.2
The practice team respects patients' rights to complain

The practice has a documented complaints policy and records all complaints and their resolution.

Criteria:

A. 5.2.1 ★ The practice team has a documented complaints policy

Interpretation

- The practice management can produce:
  - The complaints policy
  - A log of practice members who have completed training on the complaints policy
- Management can describe any ongoing or outstanding formal complaints or litigation and any previous substantive complaints or litigation which were not settled in the practice's or professional's favour

A. 5.2.2 ★ The practice team has a designated complaints officer

Interpretation

- Management and staff can identify the complaints officer

A. 5.2.3 ❄ Complaints and their resolutions are incorporated in the practice quality improvement process

Interpretation

- The practice management can produce a record of all complaints, their resolution, and any system improvements including how patients are informed of the resolution to formal complaints

Further Information (see up to date links at **http://quality.resources.machealth.ca**)

College of Physicians & Surgeons of Ontario. The Complaints Process [Internet]. [cited 2010 Jul 21]. Available from: **www.cpso.on.ca/policies/complaints/default.aspx?id=1772**

College of Nurses of Ontario. Addressing Complaints at the College of Nurses of Ontario [Internet]. 2009 Jun [cited 2010 Jul 21]. Available from: **www.cno.org/Global/docs/ih/42017_ResolvingComplaints.pdf**

Ontario College of Social Workers and Social Service Workers. Complaints [Internet]. 2010 [cited 2015 May 19]. Available from: **www.ocswssw.org/complaints-discipline/cd_complaints/**

Ontario College of Pharmacists. The Complaints Process [Internet]. 2014 [cited 2014 Jul 09]. Available from: **www.ocpinfo.com/protecting-the-public/complaints-reports/file-complaint/complaints-process/**

College of Registered Dietitians. The Jurisprudence Handbook for Dietitians in Ontario [Internet]. 2014 [cited 2015 May 19]. Available from: **www.collegeofdietitians.org/Resources/Document-Type/Jurisprudence-HandbookUpdated2014.aspx**

Pietroni PC, De Uray-Ura S. Informal complaints procedure in general practice: first year's experience. BMJ [Internet]. 1994 Jun 11[cited 2010 Jul 21];308:1546-1549. Available from: **http://bmj.bmjjournals.com/cgi/content/full/308/6943/1546**

Sub-Category A.6 Informed Decision Making

Indicator A.6.1 Patients are provided with enough information to make informed decisions about their care

Criteria

A.6.1.1 ⚖ Practice team members are trained in the CMA Code of Ethics: Communication, Decision Making and Consent

A.6.1.2 ⚖ The practice team ensures that, when required, explicit informed consent is obtained

A.6.1.3 ✻ The clinical team records advanced directives on charts

Further Information (see up to date links at **http://quality.resources.machealth.ca**)

Canadian Medical Association. Code of Ethics [Internet]. [updated 2004; cited 2014 Jul 09]. Available from: **https://www.cma.ca/Assets/assets-library/document/en/about-us/PD04-06-e.pdf**

Health Care Consent Act, 1996, S.O. 1996, c.2 Sched.A. [cited 2015 May 19]. Available from: **www.canlii.org/en/on/laws/stat/so-1996-c-2-sch-a/latest/so-1996-c-2-sch-a.html**

College of Physicians & Surgeons of Ontario. Decision-Making for the End of Life [Internet]. 2006 May/Jun/Jul [cited 2010 Jul 21]. Available from: **www.cpso.on.ca/CPSO/media/uploadedfiles/policies/policies/policyitems/End-of-Life.pdf?ext=.pdf**

Office of the Fire Marshal (Ontario). Information Bulletin – Do Not Resuscitate Confirmation Form (DNRC) [Internet]. 2008 Jan [cited 2014 Jul 09]. Available from: **www.mcscs.jus.gov.on.ca/english/FireMarshal/Forms/form_DoNotResuscitate.html**

Weston WW. Commentary: Informed and shared decision-making: the crux of patient-centred care. *CMAJ* [Internet]. 2001 Aug 21 [cited 2010 Jul 22];165(4):438-439. Available from:**www.cmaj.ca/content/165/4/438.full**

Ottawa Hospital Research Institute. Patient Decision Aids [Internet]. [cited 2010 Jul 22]. Available from: **www.ohri.ca/DecisionAid/**

Sub-Category A.6 Informed Decision Making

Indicator A.6.1
Patients are provided with enough information to make informed decisions about their care

Patients receive sufficient information and support to make informed decisions and give informed consent; appropriate forms are provided.

Criteria:

A.6.1.1 ⚖ **Practice team members are trained in the CMA Code of Ethics: Communication, Decision Making and Consent**

Interpretation

- There is a record of training of all practice team members and staff in the CMA Code of Ethics and other relevant professional codes, which includes communication, decision making and consent

A.6.1.2 ⚖ **Explicit informed consent is obtained when required**

Interpretation

- Management can produce:
  - Informed-consent forms
  - A random chart review that demonstrates the informed-consent form was completed when required
  - A patient-satisfaction questionnaire that includes a question on communication, decision making and consent

A.6.1.3 ❋ **The clinical team records advanced directives on charts**

Interpretation

- The practice management can demonstrate that:
  - Advanced-care planning is discussed with and offered to all older adult patients
  - Advanced-directives forms are available
- Management can produce the results of a random chart audit that shows advanced-directives forms have been completed

Sub-Category A.7 Educational Resources for Patients

Indicator A.7.1 The clinical team provides educational information on health promotion and prevention and disease management

Criteria

A.7.1.1 ★ A wide range of current health promotion, prevention and disease management materials is available and accessible in the practice

A.7.1.2 ❋ The clinical team provides health education

A.7.1.3 ❋ The clinical team is familiar with public health department programs

Sub-Category A.7 Educational Resources for Patients

Indicator A.7.1
The clinical team provides educational information on health promotion and prevention and disease management

Patients receive educational materials, community referrals, written and online resources and information about available public health programs.

Criteria:

A. 7.1.1 ★ A wide range of current health promotion, prevention and disease management materials is available and accessible in the practice

Interpretation

- General health promotion, prevention and disease management materials are available for patients to take home, including appropriate website addresses
- The clinical team offers patients health promotion, prevention and disease management materials, maintains those materials and ensures they are current

A.7.1.2 ❃ The clinical team provides health education

Interpretation

- The practice management can describe how the clinical team provides health education to patients (i.e., individual, group, referrals, newsletters, etc.)
- The practice can produce a list of community referral resources for education or counselling

A.7.1.3 ❃ The clinical team is familiar with public health department programs

Interpretation

- Team members can describe the programs delivered by the public health unit in their community

Further Information (see up to date links at **http://quality.resources.machealth.ca**)

College of Family Physicians of Canada. Patient Education Program [Internet]. 2007 Nov 11 [cited 2010 Jul 22]. Available from: **www.cfpc.ca/English/cfpc/programs/patient%20education/default.asp?s=1**

American Academy of Family Physicians. Health Information for the Whole Family [Internet]. 2010 [cited 2010 Jul 22]. Available from: **http://familydoctor.org/**

Ministry of Health & Long-Term Care (Ontario) Ontario Public Health Standards [Internet]. [updated 2013 Feb 22; cited 2014 Jul 09]. Available from: **www.health.gov.on.ca/en/pro/programs/publichealth/oph_standards/**

Public Health Agency of Canada. Home [Internet]. [updated 2010 Jul 20; cited 2010 Jul 22]. Available from: **www.phac-aspc.gc.ca/index-eng.php**

CATEGORY B: EQUITABLE

Indicators in this category cover equity issues: patients are accepted and treated without discrimination regardless of who they are, where they live, and when required, given extra services.

> The Institute of Medicine defines equitable as: "Providing care that does not vary in quality because of personal characteristics such as gender, ethnicity, geographic location and socioeconomic status."
>
> The Ontario Health Quality Council says: "People should get the same quality of care regardless of who they are and where they live. ... Extra help is sometimes needed to make sure everyone gets the care they need."

Category B has 1 Sub-Category with 3 Indicators

B.1 Equitable Care

Indicator B.1.1
New patients are accepted into the practice without discrimination
All clinical team members are aware of their professional obligations to accept new patients into the practice.

Indicator B.1.2
Patients get the same quality of care regardless of who they are and where they live
The quality of care is the same for all patients, including immigrants, refugees, the homeless and Aboriginal Peoples; quality is not influenced by patients' sexual orientation, gender, age, language or religion.

Indicator B.1.3
The clinical team identifies and provides additional services for patients with special needs
The clinical team can provide additional services as required for patients with special needs including cultural issues and language, impaired vision and hearing, and physical and cognitive disabilities.

Sub-Category B.1 Equitable Care

Indicator B.1.1 New patients are accepted into the practice without discrimination

Criteria

B.1.1.1 ★ All clinical team members are oriented to their regulatory college's guidelines on accepting new patients

B.1.1.2 ❃ There is a designated contact person responsible for complaints about discrimination on acceptance of new patients

Sub-Category B.1 Equitable Care

Indicator B.1.1
New patients are accepted into the practice without discrimination

All clinical team members are aware of their professional obligations to accept new patients into the practice.

Criteria:

B.1.1.1 ★ All clinical team members are oriented to their regulatory college's guidelines on accepting new patients

Interpretation

- All clinical team members have read their regulatory college's guidelines on accepting new patients (for example CPSO Guideline)

B.1.1.2 ❋ There is a designated contact person responsible for complaints about discrimination on acceptance of new patients

Interpretation

- Management and staff can identify the designated contact person responsible for complaints about discrimination against new patients
- Management documents any complaints about discrimination against new patients and their resolutions

Further Information (see up to date links at **http://quality.resources.machealth.ca**)

College of Physicians and Surgeons of Ontario. Accepting New Patients [Internet]. 2009 Apr [cited 2010 Jul 22]. Available from: **www.cpso.on.ca/policies/policies/default.aspx?ID=2506**

Sub-Category B.1 Equitable Care

Indicator B.1.2 Patients get the same quality of care regardless of who they are and where they live

Criteria

B.1.2.1 ❋ The practice team is trained to be sensitive to the needs of its practice population

B.1.2.2 ❋ There is a designated contact person responsible for complaints about discrimination

Sub-Category B.1 Equitable Care

Indicator B.1.2
Patients get the same quality of care regardless of who they are and where they live

Quality of care is the same for all patients, including immigrants, refugees, the homeless and Aboriginal Peoples; quality is not influenced by patients' sexual orientation, gender, age, language or religion.

Criteria:

B.1.2.1 ✻ **The practice team is trained to be sensitive to the needs of its practice population**

Interpretation

- Practice members are sensitized to the special needs of the practice population

B.1.2.2 ✻ **There is a designated contact person responsible for complaints about discrimination**

Interpretation

- Management and staff can identify the designated contact person responsible for complaints about discrimination
- Complaints about discrimination and their resolutions are documented

Further Information (see up to date links at **http://quality.resources.machealth.ca**)

Canadian Medical Association. Code of Ethics [Internet]. [updated 2004; cited 2014 Jul 09]. Available from: **https://www.cma.ca/Assets/assets-library/document/en/about-us/PD04-06-e.pdf**

Canadian Nurses Association. Code of Ethics for Registered Nurses – 2008 Centennial Edition [Internet]. [updated 2010 Jul 8; cited 2014 Jul 09]. Available from: **www.cna-aiic.ca/~/media/cna/files/en/codeofethics.pdf**

National Association of Social Workers (US). Code of Ethics of the National Association of Social Workers [Internet]. 2008 [cited 2010 Jul 22]. Available from: **www.socialworkers.org/pubs/code/code.asp**

Smylie J. SOGC Policy Statement: A Guide for Health Professionals Working with Aboriginal Peoples. Journal SOGC [Internet]. 2001 Jan [cited 2015 May 19].;1-15. Available from: **www.cfpc.ca/uploadedFiles/Resources/Resource_Items/Health_Professionals/GuideHealthProfessionalsAboriginal.pdf**

Society of Obstetricians and Gynaecologists of Canada. SOGC Guidelines: Aboriginal Guidelines [Internet]. [updated 2010 Jun 29; cited 2010 Jul 22]. Available from: **www.sogc.org/guidelines/index_e.asp#aboriginal**

Canadian Medical Association. Code of Ethics [Internet]. [updated 2004; cited 2014 Jul 09]. Available from: **https://www.cma.ca/Assets/assets-library/document/en/about-us/PD04-06-e.pdf**

Ontario Council of Agencies Serving Immigrants. Health [Internet]. 2010 [cited 2010 Jul 22]. Available from: **www.settlement.org/topics.asp?section=HE**

Sub-Category B.1 Equitable Care

Indicator B.1.3 The clinical team identifies and provides additional services for patients with special needs

Criteria	B.1.3.1	❋	The clinical team can identify patients with special needs who require additional services
	B.1.3.2	❋	The clinical team has links to community groups that can help it provide additional services to patients with special needs

Sub-Category B.1 Equitable Care

Indicator B.1.3
The clinical team identifies and provides additional services for patients with special needs

The clinical team can provide additional services as required for patients with special needs including cultural issues and language, impaired vision and hearing, and physical and cognitive disabilities.

Criteria:

B.1.3.1 ❋ The clinical team can identify patients with special needs who require additional services

Interpretation

- The practice management can demonstrate that:
  - The patient's chart highlights special needs and additional services required (such as cultural issues or language, hearing or vision impairment, cognitive disabilities, etc.)
  - The booking system can identify additional services required (such as translators, communication tools for hearing-impaired and blind patients, accompaniment by family/caregivers for physical and cognitive disabilities, etc.)
  - All clinical team members can access a record of additional services required for out-of-office and/or after-hours care
  - Every patient chart lists the patient's first language, whether there is a barrier to communication that requires a translator and who to use

B. 1.3.2 ❋ The clinical team has links to community groups that can help it provide additional services to patients with special needs

Interpretation

- The practice management can provide a list of community groups that provide additional services to patients with special needs

Further Information (see up to date links at **http://quality.resources.machealth.ca**)

Canadian Medical Association. Code of Ethics [Internet]. [updated 2004; cited 2014 Jul 09]. Available from: **https://www.cma.ca/Assets/assets-library/document/en/about-us/PD04-06-e.pdf**

Ontario Association of the Deaf. Welcome to the Ontario Association of the Deaf [Internet]. [cited 2010 Jul 22]. Available from: **www.deafontario.ca/**

Ontario Human Rights Commission. Disability and the Duty to Accommodate: Your Rights and Responsibilities [Internet]. 2008 [updated 2010 Jul 20; cited 2010 Jul 21]. Available from: **www.ohrc.on.ca/en/issues/disability**

Canadian National Institute for the Blind. Our Services [Internet]. [cited 2014 Jul 09]. Available from: **www.cnib.ca/en/services/Pages/default.aspx**

CATEGORY C: TIMELY AND ACCESSIBLE

Indicators in this category cover issues of timeliness and accessibility: Patients receive appointments, referrals, test results and after-hours or emergency care in a timely manner, and new patients' medical records are transferred efficiently.

The Institute of Medicine defines timely as: "Reducing waits and sometimes harmful delays for both those who receive and those who give care."

The Ontario Health Quality Council defines accessible as: "Getting the right care at the right time in the right setting by the right health-care provider."

Category C has 2 Sub-Categories with 6 Indicators

C.1 Timely and Accessible

Indicator C.1.1

Patients can reach the practice by telephone, email and/or other electronic means

Telephone system, email and/or other electronic systems are user-friendly and facilitate easy access to the practice.

Indicator C.1.2

Patients can book appropriate appointments

Patients can book longer or shorter appointments as needed and wait-times are monitored.

Indicator C.1.3

Registration of new patients and transfer of medical records are timely and accessible

New patients are registered efficiently and their medical records are transferred to and from the practice according to CPSO guidelines.

Indicator C.1.4

Investigations and referrals occur in a timely manner

There is a system in place to monitor wait times for investigations and referrals.

C.2 After-Hours and Emergency Care

Indicator C.2.1

The clinical team provides access to 24-hour care, seven days a week

The practice ensures access to 24/7 medical care; alternative arrangements are provided if the clinical team does not provide 24-hour care.

Indicator C.2.2

The practice team responds to emergencies/ urgent medical conditions

Patients are able to book urgent-care visits; the practice team is trained to recognize and respond to emergencies.

Sub-Category C.1 Timely and Accessible

Indicator C.1.1 Patients can reach the practice by telephone, email and/or other electronic means

Criteria C.1.1.1 ✻ There is an effective telephone system, email and/or other electronic system for booking appointments, getting advice and leaving messages

Sub-Category C.1 Timely and Accessible

Indicator C.1.1
Patients can access the practice using the telephone system, email and/or other electronic means

The telephone system, email and/or other electronic systems are user-friendly and facilitate easy access to the practice.

Criteria:

C.1.1.1 ❋ There is an effective telephone system, email and/or other electronic means for booking appointments, getting advice and leaving messages

Interpretation

- Management can describe:
  - The telephone system (incoming and outgoing calls) and voice-mail messaging system and how it responds
  - The email and/or other electronic system used for communications with patients
  - How patients can obtain advice or information related to their clinical care without an appointment (e.g., by telephone or electronic means)
  - How feedback from patients is sought and used to make changes to the phone or message system (e.g., through an annual patient satisfaction survey)
- The practice conducts a regular telephone audit of incoming calls, number of rings to answer, time left on hold, and callbacks, including how messages are recorded, retrieved and followed up

Further Information (see up to date links at **http://quality.resources.machealth.ca**)

College of Physicians & Surgeons of Ontario. Medical Records [Internet]. 2006 Mar/Apr. Chapter 5, Procedural Medicine – Telephone Conversation and Emails. [cited 2010 Jul 21].
Available from: **www.cpso.on.ca/policies/policies/default.aspx?id=1686&terms=privacy+and+record+keeping**

Howard M, Agarwal G, Hilts L. Patient satisfaction with access in two interprofessional academic family medicine clinics. Family Practice [Internet]. 2009 Oct [cited 2010 Jul 22];26(5):407-412.
Available from: **http://fampra.oxfordjournals.org/cgi/content/abstract/26/5/407** DOI:10.1093/fampra/cmp049

Hallam L. Organisation of telephone services and patients' access to doctors by telephone in general practice. BMJ [Internet]. 1991 Mar 16 [cited 2010 Jul 22];302(6777):629-32.
Available from: **www.ncbi.nlm.nih.gov/entrez/query.fcgi?cmd=Retrieve&db=PubMed&list_uids=2012879&dopt=Abstract**

de Groot RA, de Haan J, Bosveld HEP, Nijland A, Meyboom-de Jong B. The implementation of a call-back system reduces the doctor's workload, and improves accessibility by telephone in general practice. Family Practice [Internet]. 2002 [cited 2010 Jul 22];19(5):516-519.
Available from: **http://fampra.oupjournals.org/cgi/content/abstract/19/5/516**

Sub-Category C.1 Timely and Accessible

Indicator C.1.2 Patients can book appropriate appointments

Criteria

C.1.2.1 ❋ Patients can book regular, longer or shorter appointments if necessary

C.1.2.2 ❋ The practice team monitors wait-times for appointments

C.1.2.3 ❋ The clinical team endeavours to be on time for patient visits

Sub-Category C.1 Timely and Accessible

Indicator C.1.2
Patients can book appropriate appointments

Patients can book longer or shorter appointments as needed and wait-times are monitored.

Criteria:

C.1.2.1 ❋ **Patients can book regular, longer or shorter appointments if necessary**

Interpretation

- The booking system accommodates longer or shorter appointments according to clinical need
- An annual patient-satisfaction survey shows that patients are satisfied with the length of their appointments

C.1.2.2 ❋ **The practice team monitors wait-times for appointments**

Interpretation

- Management monitors the wait-time to the next available appointment (the "third next available appointment" system or an equivalent can be used to measure delay)

C.1.2.3 ❋ **The clinical team endeavours to be on time for patient visits**

Interpretation

- An annual patient satisfaction survey shows that patients are satisfied with the timeliness of their appointments
- An annual audit measures the ratio between wait-time and visit (e.g., the optimal ratio is 1:3 to 2:3)

Further Information (see up to date links at **http://quality.resources.machealth.ca**)

College of Physicians & Surgeons of Ontario. Medical Records [Internet]. 2006 Mar/Apr. Chapter 2, Overview and Organization of Medical Records – The Daily Diary of Appointments. [cited 2010 Jul 21]. Available from: **www.cpso.on.ca/policies/policies/default.aspx?id=1686**

Murray M, Tantau C. Same-Day Appointments: Exploding the Access Paradigm. Family Practice Management [Internet]. 2000 [cited 2010 Jul 22]. Available from: **www.aafp.org/fpm/20000900/45same.html**

Institute for Healthcare Improvement. Third Next Available Appointment [Internet]. [cited 2010 Jul 22]. Available from: **www.ihi.org/knowledge/Pages/Measures/ThirdNextAvailableAppointment.aspx**

Howard M, Agarwal G, Hilts L. Patient satisfaction with access in two interprofessional academic family medicine clinics. Family Practice [Internet]. 2009 Oct [cited 2010 Jul 22];26(5):407-412. Available from: **http://fampra.oxfordjournals.org/cgi/content/abstract/26/5/407** DOI:10.1093/fampra/cmp049

Sub-Category C.1 Timely and Accessible

Indicator C.1.3 Registration of new patients and transfer of medical records are timely and accessible

Criteria

C.1.3.1 ❋ There is a patient registration process for collecting personal and health information that is timely, efficient and patient-friendly

C.1.3.2 ★ Details of the transfer of medical records to and from the practice are recorded according to CPSO guidelines

Sub-Category C.1 Timely and Accessible

Indicator C.1.3
Registration of new patients and transfer of medical records are timely and accessible

New patients are registered efficiently and their medical records are transferred to and from the practice according to CPSO guidelines.

Criteria:

C.1.3.1 ❋ The patient registration process for collecting personal and health information is timely, efficient and patient-friendly

Interpretation

- Management can describe how the registration process is timely, efficient and patient-friendly

C.1.3.2 ★ Details of the transfer of medical records to and from the practice are recorded according to CPSO guidelines

Interpretation

- New patients' written consent to access their previous medical records is obtained
- Medical records are transferred in a timely manner
- The transferred records are documented and include: copy of request, name and address of requesting physician, date of transfer, method of transfer, copy of summary sent

Further Information (see up to date links at **http://quality.resources.machealth.ca**)

College of Physicians & Surgeons of Ontario. Medical Records [Internet]. 2006 Mar/Apr [cited 2010 Jul 21]. Available from: **www.cpso.on.ca/policies/policies/default.aspx?id=1686**

Ministry of Health & Long-term Care (Ontario). Health Information Protection Act, 2004 [Internet]. 2002 [updated 2012 Jun 25; cited 2014 Jul 09]. Available from: **www.health.gov.on.ca/en/common/legislation/priv_legislation/**

Canadian Medical Protective Association. A Matter of Records: Retention and Transfer of Clinical Records. CMPA [Internet]. 2003 [revised 2008; cited 2014 Jul 09].;1-4. Available from: **https://oplfrpd5.cmpa-acpm.ca/en/duties-and-responsibilities/-/asset_publisher/bFaUiyQG069N/content/a-matter-of-records-retention-and-transfer-of-clinical-records**

Sub-Category C.1 Timely and Accessible

Indicator C.1.4 Investigations and referrals occur in a timely manner

Criteria C.1.4.1 ★ Patients are referred promptly for both investigations and referrals

Sub-Category C.1 Timely and Accessible

Indicator C.1.4
Investigations and referrals occur in a timely manner

There is a system in place to monitor wait times for investigations and referrals.

Criteria:

C.1.4.1 ★ Patients are referred promptly for both investigations and referrals

Interpretation

- The practice team monitors referrals and investigations according to national and local guidelines and procedures
- The results of the annual patient satisfaction survey show that patients are satisfied with the referral system for investigations and consultations
- An annual chart audit monitors wait times to referral for investigations and consults

Further Information (see up to date links at **http://quality.resources.machealth.ca**)

Canadian Medical Protective Association. Wait Times - A Medical Liability Perspective [Internet]. [cited 2014 Jul 09]. Available from: **https://oplfrpd5.cmpa-acpm.ca/en/public-policy/-/asset_publisher/9rnAcJbTAZA6/content/wait-times-a-medical-liability-perspective**

Canadian Medical Protective Association. Failure to make the diagnosis of colorectal cancer: A window of opportunity missed [Internet]. 2008 Sept [cited 2014 Jul 09]. Available from: **https://oplfrpd5.cmpa-acpm.ca/en/safety/-/asset_publisher/N6oEDMrzRbCC/content/failure-to-make-the-diagnosis-of-colorectal-cancer-a-window-of-opportunity-missed**

College of Physicians & Surgeons of Ontario. Practice Assessment Report – Continuity of Care and Referrals [Internet]. 2008 Mar 18 [cited 2010 Jul 22]. Available from: **www.cpso.on.ca/uploadedFiles/downloads/cpsodocuments/members/peerassessment/Continuity.pdf**

College of Physicians & Surgeons of Ontario.Test Results Management [Internet]. 2011 Feb [cited 2014 Jul 14]. Avalable from: **www.cpso.on.ca/CPSO/media/uploadedfiles/policies/policies/policyitems/test_results.pdf?ext=.pdf**

Sub-Category C.2 After-Hours and Emergency Care

Indicator C.2.1 The clinical team provides access to 24-hour care, seven days a week

Criteria

- C.2.1.1 ★ Information is available about how the practice provides 24-hour medical coverage (⚖ for PCNs, FHNs, special contracts)
- C.2.1.2 ★ Patients can reach the after-hours service by telephone
- C.2.1.3 ❋ The on-call physician can access core patient information – Cumulative Patient Profile (CPP)
- C.2.1.4 ❋ A record of patients' after-hours visits to the on-call service is sent to the patients' physician (⚖ for PCNs, FHNs, special contracts with Telehealth Ontario)

Sub-Category C.2 After-Hours and Emergency Care

Indicator C.2.1
The clinical team provides access to 24-hour care, seven days a week

The practice ensures access to 24/7 medical care; alternative arrangements are provided if the clinical team does not provide 24-hour care.

Criteria:

C.2.1.1 ★ Information is available about how the practice provides 24-hour medical coverage (⚖ for PCNs, FHNs, special contracts)

Interpretation

- The practice posts clear information on how patients can access 24-hour care, e.g., in a brochure, pamphlet, or on a website
- Management can describe how the clinical team provides 24-hour care (e.g., regular office hours, extended hours, on-call services, telephone access and other services, such as Telehealth)

C.2.1.2 ★ Patients can reach the after-hours service via telephone

Interpretation

- An annual audit monitors the practice's after-hours telephone system (e.g., can patients reach care with two calls?)
- The annual patient satisfaction survey includes after-hours care

C.2.1.3 ❃ The on-call physician can access core patient information – Cumulative Patient Profile (CPP)

Interpretation

- There is a way for the on-call physician to access patients' CPP (in accordance with privacy legislation Bill 31)

C.2.1.4 ❃ A record of patients' after-hours visits to the on-call service is sent to the patients' physician (⚖ for PCNs, FHNs, special contracts with Telehealth Ontario)

Interpretation

- The practice management can provide a sample of on-call information sent in a timely manner from the after-hours service during the previous week
- The practice has a system to manage non-registered patients seen after-hours

Further Information (see up to date links at **http://quality.resources.machealth.ca**)

College of Physicians & Surgeons of Ontario. Medical Records [Internet]. 2006 Mar/Apr. Chapter 3, General Principles for Contents of Medical Records – The Cumulative Patient Profile. [cited 2010 Jul 21]. Available from: **www.cpso.on.ca/policies/policies/default.aspx?id=1686**

College of Physicians & Surgeons of Ontario. Practice Assessment Report – Record Keeping and Patient Management Tools [Internet]. 2008 Mar 18 [cited 2010 Jul 22]. Available from: **www.cpso.on.ca/uploadedFiles/downloads/cpsodocuments/members/peerassessment/RecordKeepingTOOL.pdf**

Ministry of Health and Long-Term Care (Ontario). Public Information - Telehealth Ontario [Internet]. 2009 Aug 17 [cited 2010 Jul 22]. Available from: **www.health.gov.on.ca/en/public/programs/telehealth/**

Sub-Category C.2 After-Hours and Emergency Care

Indicator C.2.2 The practice team responds to emergencies and urgent medical conditions

Criteria	C.2.2.1	★	Patients are able to book urgent-care visits
	C.2.2.2	❋	All members of the practice team are trained to recognize and respond to emergencies and urgent medical conditions
	C.2.2.3	❋	The reception team/person can reach a relevant clinical team member if immediate attention is required
	C.2.2.4	❋	Members of the practice team have current CPR/BCLS certificates

Sub-Category C.2 After-Hours and Emergency Care

Indicator C.2.2
The practice team responds to emergencies and urgent medical conditions

Patients are able to book urgent-care visits; the practice team is trained to recognize and respond to emergencies.

Criteria:

C.2.2.1 ★ Patients are able to book urgent-care visits

Interpretation

- Patients can book urgent-care visits (urgent care is medical care for a condition that is not an emergency but is severe or painful enough to require treatment or evaluation within a reasonable period of time in order to avoid serious deterioration of the patient's condition or health)
- There is a system for monitoring the availability of urgent-care appointments
- The annual patient satisfaction survey includes urgent-care appointments

C.2.2.2 ❋ All members of the practice team are trained to recognize and respond to emergencies and urgent medical conditions

Interpretation

- The practice team is prepared to recognize and respond to emergencies and urgent medical conditions
- The annual audit includes the records of patients with emergencies and urgent medical conditions

C.2.2.3 ❋ The reception team/person can reach a relevant clinical team member if immediate attention is required

Interpretation

- The reception team can reach an appropriate clinical team member to assist patients who need urgent attention

C.2.2.4 ❋ Members of the practice team have current CPR/BCLS certificates

Interpretation

- Management can produce a record of current CPR/BCLS certificates

Further Information (see up to date links at **http://quality.resources.machealth.ca**)

Heart and Stroke Foundation of Ontario. Heart and Stroke for Healthcare Professionals [Internet]. 2010 [cited 2010 Jul 22]. Available from: **www.heartandstroke.com/site/c.ikIQLcMWJtE/b.3856593/k.B76E/For_Professionals.htm**

CATEGORY D: SAFE

Indicators in this category cover safety issues: infection control, vaccine storage, office procedures, disposal of sharps and medical waste, safe and appropriate medical equipment, drug and prescription management, medical record storage, ensuring essential information is included in medical records, tracking test results and incident reporting.

> The Institute of Medicine defines safe as:
> "Avoiding injuries to patients from the care that is intended to help them."
> (Do no harm.)
>
> The Ontario Health Quality Council says:
> "People should not be harmed by an accident or mistakes when they receive care."

Category D has 8 Sub-Categories with 11 Indicators

D.1 Infection Control

Indicator D.1.1

The practice team follows infection-control guidelines

Team members follow disinfection and sterilization guidelines, store sterile instruments appropriately and practise hand hygiene.

D.2 Cold Chain

Indicator D.2.1

The practice team follows provincial guidelines for vaccine storage/cold chain

Guidelines for effective vaccine storage include using a designated refrigerator and ensuring that vaccines are current.

D.3 Office Procedures

Indicator D.3.1

Procedures performed in the office conform to accepted guidelines

The practice has a list of approved procedures, and clinical team members have suitable training and equipment to perform these procedures in accordance with accepted guidelines.

D.4 Disposal of Sharps and Biomedical Waste

Indicator D.4.1

The practice team safely disposes of sharps and biomedical waste

The practice team has a system to safely dispose of sharps and contaminated materials.

D.5 Medical Equipment

Indicator D.5.1

Medical equipment and resources are safe, appropriate, secure, available and maintained

The practice's medical equipment is safe, appropriate, available when required, and well-maintained.

D.6 Drugs

Indicator D.6.1

Drugs available in the practice are appropriate, controlled, secure and maintained

Recommended steps for controlling drugs in the practice include authorized access, secure storage, a bi-annual audit, and dispensing records.

Indicator D.6.2

Prescription management

Medications ordered for patients are prescribed and managed in the safest manner possible.

D.7 Medical Record-keeping

Indicator D.7.1
Medical records are stored or filed safely and securely

Steps to ensure that medical records are stored securely and retrievable only by authorized medical staff include safe storage of backup tapes or CDs, computer password protection and lockouts, and an IT strategic plan.

Indicator D.7.2
Medical records include all essential information necessary to provide quality patient care

Patient records should include cumulative patient profiles, up-to-date lists of problems and medications, telephone conversations, clinical decisions and all other necessary information about the patient and their care in accordance with best-practice guidelines, legal and local standards.

Indicator D.7.3
There is a system to track and manage patient test results and medical reports

The practice has an effective system in place for managing test results and medical reports, including follow-up of missing results and notification of patients.

D.8 Incident Reporting

Indicator D.8.1
There is an incident reporting system to identify and address serious or potentially serious adverse events

An incident reporting and management system is in place that identifies and addresses adverse events, errors, near-misses, etc.

Sub-Category D.1 Infection Control

Indicator D.1.1 The practice team follows infection-control guidelines

Criteria

- **D.1.1.1** ⚖ There is a procedure for infection control
- **D.1.1.2** ⚖ Hand hygiene is practised throughout the practice
- **D.1.1.3** ⚖ The practice team cleans and disinfects equipment and facilities
- **D.1.1.4** ⚖ The practice team sterilizes instruments and materials
- **D.1.1.5** ⚖ Sterile or surgically clean instruments are stored to ensure sterility
- **D.1.1.6** ⚖ Practice team members are trained in cleaning, disinfecting and sterilizing equipment

Sub-Category D.1 Infection Control

Indicator D.1.1
The practice team follows infection-control guidelines

Team members follow disinfection and sterilization guidelines, store sterile instruments appropriately and practise hand hygiene.

Criteria

D.1.1.1 ⚖ There is a procedure for infection control

Interpretation

- The practice has procedures for infection control that follow recent guidelines (pandemic planning for H1N1, SARS, etc.)
- The practice team monitors and reviews infection-control procedures
- There is a bi-annual audit of various infection-control procedures, including human resources, hand hygiene, instruments and office equipment/ furniture, and waste management

D.1.1.2 ⚖ Hand hygiene is practised throughout the practice

Interpretation

- The practice has facilities for handwashing in all clinical management areas (Low- and medium-risk handwashing facilities should include liquid soap and water, disposable paper towels or single-use towels. Reusable cloth towels, if used at all, should not be used in treatment areas or toilets and they should be changed frequently)
- Where a hand basin is not available (for example during off-site visits), waterless hand scrubs or alcohol preparations are available
- The practice team promotes frequent handwashing
- Sterile handwashing with liquid soap and water is practised before surgical procedures

D.1.1.3 ⚖ The practice team cleans and disinfects equipment and facilities

Interpretation

- Team members clean and disinfect equipment and facilities routinely, clean and disinfect blood and body-substance spills, and clean all instruments, including those off-site
- Members clean and/or dispose of low-risk and single-use instruments/ equipment and linen

Indicator D.1.1
The practice team follows infection-control guidelines *(continued)*

D.1.1.4 ⚖ The practice team sterilizes instruments and materials

Interpretation

The practice management can describe how the practice team:

- Sterilizes instruments and materials (all types of sterilization equipment used in the practice)
- Monitors, validates, maintains and calibrates sterilization equipment
- Uses disposable instruments
- Avoids sterilization environmental hazards (e.g., gluteraldehyde, WHMIS)

D.1.1.5 ⚖ Sterile or surgically clean instruments are stored to ensure sterility

Interpretation

- The practice team stores sterile or surgically clean instruments in a protected area (e.g., a closed cupboard, sealed containers, etc.)
- There is a dating rotation system for packaged surgical instruments

D.1.1.6 ⚖ Practice team members are trained in cleaning, disinfecting and sterilizing equipment

Interpretation

- Management can identify:
  - The practice team member(s) trained in disinfection and sterilization
  - The person responsible for infection control for the practice
  - The person responsible for sterilization procedures for the practice

Further Information (see up to date links at **http://quality.resources.machealth.ca**)

College of Physicians and Surgeons of Ontario. Infection Control in the Physician's Office [Internet]. 2004 [cited 2010 Jul 22]. Available from: **www.cpso.on.ca/policies-publications/cpgs-other-guidelines/other-guidelines/infection-prevention-and-control-for-clinical-offi**

Canadian Centre for Occupational Health and Safety. Nurse (Registered) [Internet]. 2003 Mar 27 [cited 2010 Jul 22]. Available from: **www.ccohs.ca/oshanswers/occup_workplace/nurse.html**

Hellekson K. Practice Guidelines: AAP Issues Recommendations on Infection Control in Physicians' Offices. Am Fam Physician [Internet]. 2001 Feb 15 [cited 2010 Jul 22];63(4):787-789. Available from: **www.aafp.org/afp/2001/0215/p787.html**

Health Canada. Workplace Hazardous Materials Information System [Internet]. [updated 2010 Jul 10; cited 2010 Jul 22]. Available from: **www.hc-sc.gc.ca/ewh-semt/occup-travail/whmis-simdut/index-eng.php**

Ministry of Health and Long-Term Care (Ontario). H1N1 Flu Virus: Health Care Professionals [Internet]. [updated 2010 Jun 17; cited 2010 Jul 22]. Available from: **www.health.gov.on.ca/english/providers/program/emu/ihn.html**

Sub-Category D.2 Cold Chain

Indicator D.2.1 The practice team follows provincial guidelines for vaccine storage/cold chain

Criteria

D.2.1.1 ⚖ There is a designated vaccine refrigerator

D.2.1.2 ⚖ A daily log shows effective monitoring of the fridge temperature

D.2.1.3 ⚖ Vaccines are current

D.2.1.4 ⚖ National/provincial guidelines are used to preserve the cold chain during office and off-site immunizations

Further Information (see up to date links at **http://quality.resources.machealth.ca**)

College of Physicians and Surgeons of Ontario. A Practical Guide for Safe and Effective Office-Based Practices [Internet]. 2012 May [cited 2014 Jul 09].
Available from: **www.cpso.on.ca/uploadedFiles/policies/guidelines/office/Safe-Practices.pdf**

Public Health Agency of Canada. National Vaccine Storage and Handling Guidelines for Immunization Providers [Internet]. 2007 [updated 2007 Dec 14; cited 2010 Jul 22].
Available from: **www.phac-aspc.gc.ca/publicat/2007/nvshglp-ldemv/section1-eng.php**

Toronto Public Health. Fact Sheet: Vaccine Storage and Handling - The Cold Chain Program [Internet]. 2008 Jun [cited 2010 Jul 22].
Available from: **www.toronto.ca/health/professionals/immunization/cold_chain.htm**

Public Health Agency of Canada: Canadian Immunization Guide. [cited 2015 Oct 08].
Available from **www.phac-aspc.gc.ca/publicat/cig-gci/index-eng.php**

Sub-Category D.2 Cold Chain

Indicator D.2.1
The practice team follows provincial guidelines for vaccine storage/cold chain

Guidelines for effective vaccine storage include using a designated refrigerator and ensuring that vaccines are current.

Criteria

D.2.1.1 ⚖ There is a designated vaccine refrigerator

Interpretation

- There is a designated vaccine fridge that does not contain anything other than vaccine-related substances (i.e., no food, drinks or specimens)

D.2.1.2 ⚖ A daily log shows effective monitoring of the fridge temperature

Interpretation

- The vaccine-fridge log includes a record of the daily date, time, temperature and any action taken to correct abnormal readings
- There is a minimum/maximum thermometer or electronic probe in the fridge
- There is a person responsible for monitoring the daily log and maintaining the fridge (e.g., electronic thermometer and temperatures)
- There is a record that shows all members of the team know the guidelines for vaccine storage/cold chain

D.2.1.3 ⚖ Vaccines are current

Interpretation

- There is a procedure to ensure all vaccine expiry dates are current (e.g., random sample of stocks)
- A dating rotation system is used to keep vaccines current (i.e., stock rotation, ordering, proper storage)

D.2.1.4 ⚖ National/provincial guidelines are used to preserve the cold chain during office and off-site immunizations

Interpretation

- There is a procedure to preserve the cold chain while in the office and during transport for off-site immunizations
- There is a contingency plan for a cold-chain incident or a power failure

Sub-Category D.3 Office Procedures

Indicator D.3.1 Procedures performed in the office conform to accepted guidelines

Criteria

D.3.1.1 ★ There is a list of approved procedures performed in the practice

D.3.1.2 ★ Clinical team members are trained to perform the listed procedures

D.3.1.3 ★ The practice has appropriate equipment and facilities for the procedures

D.3.1.4 ★ Patients who require procedures sign consent forms

D.3.1.5 ❃ Clinical team members keep a record or log of their procedures

Further Information (see up to date links at **http://quality.resources.machealth.ca**)

Ministry of Health and Long-Term Care (Ontario). Bulletin 4395: Physician Supervision of Simple Office Procedures [Internet]. [updated 2009 Jun 15; cited 2014 Jul 09].
Available from: **www.health.gov.on.ca/en/pro/programs/ohip/bulletins/4395/bul4395.aspx**

College of Physicians and Surgeons of Ontario. A Practical Guide for Safe and Effective Office-Based Practices [Internet]. 2009 Apr [cited 2014 Jul 09].
Available from: **www.cpso.on.ca/uploadedFiles/policies/guidelines/office/Safe-Practices.pdf**

An Interprofessional guide on the Use of Orders, Directives and Delegation for Regulated Health Professionals in Ontario. Frequently Asked Questions. [Internet]. 2007 [cited 2014 Jul 9].
Available from: **http://mdguide.regulatedhealthprofessions.on.ca/why/faq/default.asp#faq01**

Sub-Category D.3 Office Procedures

Indicator D.3.1
Procedures performed in the office conform to accepted guidelines

The practice has a list of approved procedures, and clinical team members have suitable training and equipment to perform these procedures in accordance with accepted guidelines.

Criteria

D.3.1.1 ★ There is a list of approved procedures performed in the practice

Interpretation

- Management has a list of all procedures that can be performed in the office

D.3.1.2 ★ Clinical team members are trained to perform the listed procedures

Interpretation

- Management can provide an annually updated list of the clinical team members approved to perform each office procedure

D.3.1.3 ★ The practice has appropriate equipment and facilities for the procedures

Interpretation

- The practice annually (or more frequently) monitors its equipment and facilities required for the procedures

D.3.1.4 ★ Patients who require procedures sign consent forms

Interpretation

- Patients are offered information and choice about all procedures to be performed in the practice (See also Indicator A.6.1: Patients are provided with enough information to make informed decisions about their care)
- A random chart audit shows that consent was signed for appropriate procedures

D.3.1.5 ❃ Clinical team members keep a record or log of their procedures

Interpretation

- The practice's record or log of procedures includes:
  - Date of procedure
  - Patient name
  - Procedure performed
  - Whether a specimen was sent for pathology
  - Date result received
  - Date patient was informed of result

Sub-Category D.4 Disposal of Sharps and Biomedical Waste

Indicator D.4.1 The practice team safely disposes of sharps and biomedical waste

Criteria

D.4.1.1 ⚖ Biomedical waste is safely stored and disposed of in accordance with local regulations (including anatomical waste, blood, non-anatomical waste and other waste material)

D.4.1.2 ⚖ The practice has appropriate puncture-resistant sharps containers with a biohazard symbol, placed in all areas where sharps are used

D.4.1.3 ⚖ The practice team has a protocol/policy and procedures in case of an accidental needle-stab or other type of exposure

Sub-Category D.4 Disposal of Sharps and Biomedical Waste

Indicator D.4.1
The practice team safely disposes of sharps and biomedical waste

The practice team has a system to safely dispose of sharps and contaminated materials.

Criteria:

D.4.1.1 ⚖ **Biomedical waste is safely stored and disposed of in accordance with local regulations (including anatomical waste, blood, non-anatomical waste and other waste material)**

Interpretation

- There is a plan for disposal of biomedical waste
- The practice team stores biomedical waste safely (e.g., in a closed cupboard or sealed plastic container)
- The disposal of biomedical waste meets local regulations (All waste must be collected and transported by a waste management company that is licensed to transport biomedical waste. This waste must be packaged and colour-coded according to your agreement with your biomedical waste contractor)

D.4.1.2 ⚖ **The practice has appropriate puncture-resistant sharps containers with a biohazard symbol, placed in all areas where sharps are used**

Interpretation

- Puncture-resistant sharps containers must be visible in clinical areas where sharps are used, display a biohazard symbol, and be mounted securely
- Sharps containers must be placed out of the reach of children

D.4.1.3 ⚖ **The practice team has a protocol/policy and procedures in case of an accidental needle-stab or other type of exposure**

Interpretation

- The practice has protocols for:
  - Managing accidental needle-stab injuries
  - Documenting all accidental needle-stab injuries
  - Managing other types of exposure or injuries
  - Documenting other exposure or injuries

Further Information (see up to date links at **http://quality.resources.machealth.ca**)

Alberta Medical Association. Managing Office Biomedical Waste [Internet] . 2014 [cited 2014 Jul 09]. Available from: **https://www.albertadoctors.org/leaders-partners/quality-and-education-programs/clinical-resources/biomedical-waste**

Canadian Centre for Occupational Health and Safety. Needlestick Injuries [Internet]. [updated 2005 Jan 25; cited 2010 Jul 22]. Available from: **www.ccohs.ca/oshanswers/diseases/needlestick_injuries.html**

Health Canada. Workplace Hazardous Materials Information System [Internet]. [updated 2010 Jul 10; cited 2010 Jul 22]. Available from: **www.hc-sc.gc.ca/ewh-semt/occup-travail/whmis-simdut/index-eng.php**

Sub-Category D.5 Medical Equipment

Indicator D.5.1 Medical equipment and resources are safe, appropriate, secure, available and maintained

Criteria

D.5.1.1 ★ Medical equipment is safe, appropriate, secure and maintained in good working order

D.5.1.2 ★ All essential emergency equipment is safe, available and maintained in good working order

Further Information (see up to date links at **http://quality.resources.machealth.ca**)

College of Physicians and Surgeons of Ontario. A Practical Guide for Safe and Effective Office-Based Practices [Internet]. 2009 Apr [cited 2014 Jul 09].
Available from: **www.cpso.on.ca/uploadedFiles/policies/guidelines/office/Safe-Practices.pdf**

Sempowski IP, Brison RJ. Dealing with office emergencies: Stepwise approach for family physicians. CFP [Internet]. 2002 Sept [cited 2010 Jul 22]. Available from: **www.cfp.ca/content/48/9/1464.abstract**

Paediatric emergency equipment and supplies: Guidelines for physician's offices. CFP [Internet]. 2001 Apr [cited 2010 Jul 22];47:797-799. Available from: **www.ncbi.nlm.nih.gov/pmc/articles/PMC2735386/**

Royal New Zealand College of General Practitioners. Aiming for Excellence – An Assessment Tool for New Zealand General Practice. 3rd ed [monograph online]. New Zealand: Royal New Zealand College of General Practitioners (RNZCGP); 2009. Indicator B.5.1, Medical equipment and resources are available and maintained; p.46-48. [cited 2010 Jul 22].
Available from: **www.rnzcgp.org.nz/assets/documents/CORNERSTONE/Aiming-for-Excellence-2009-including-record-review.pdf**

Friesen K. Ontario's Role in National Mercury Elimination and Reduction Strategy [Internet]. Pollution Probe; 2008 Mar 3 [cited 2015 Oct 08].
Available from: **http://books1.scholarsportal.info/viewdoc.html?id=/ebooks/ebooks0/gibson_cppc/2009-12-01/10/252171**

Environment Canada. Risk Management Strategy for Mercury-Containing Products. CEPA Environmental Registry [Internet]. [updated 2006 Dec 20; cited 2010 Jul 22].
Available from: **www.ec.gc.ca/ceparegistry/documents/part/Merc_RMS/Merc_RMS.cfm#4**

Environment Canada. Cleaning up small mercury spills [Internet]. [updated 2010 Apr 26; cited 2010 Jul 22].
Available from: **www.ec.gc.ca/mercure-mercury/default.asp?lang=En&n=D2B2AD47-1**

Sub-Category D.5 Medical Equipment

Indicator D.5.1
Medical equipment in the practice is safe, appropriate, secure, available and maintained

The practice's medical equipment is safe, appropriate, available when required, and well-maintained.

Criteria:

D.5.1.1 ★ Medical equipment is safe, appropriate, secure and maintained in good working order

Interpretation

- The practice management maintains a list of all medical equipment
- An annual audit of medical equipment (which includes confirmation that the equipment was appropriate, safe and maintained in good working order) is conducted. The following basic office equipment if available should be in good working order:
  - Thermometers*
  - Sphygmomanometer – calibrated within the past year*
  - Stethoscope
  - Otoscope/Ophthalmoscope
  - Tendon hammer
  - Peak flow meter (both adult and pediatric)
  - Tape measure
  - Weighing scales
  - Height measure
  - Snellen chart
  - Tuning fork
  - Urine testing sticks – check expiry dates
  - Vaginal specula
  - Foetal Doppler
  - Fridge min/max thermometer
  - Suction
  - Equipment for procedures (e.g., sutures, biopsies, IUDs, circumcisions, etc.)
  - Other equipment as needed to accommodate the office practices and procedures
- Syringes, needles and other equipment that might be stolen is not visible in examining rooms

D.5.1.2 ★ All essential emergency equipment is safe, available and maintained in good working order

Interpretation

- The practice management maintains a list of all emergency equipment
- A quarterly audit of emergency equipment includes confirmation that the equipment is appropriate, safe and maintained in good working order

* No mercury-containing thermometers or sphygmomanometers

Sub-Category D.6 Drugs

Indicator D.6.1 Drugs used in the practice are appropriate, controlled, secure and maintained

Criteria

D.6.1.1 ★ There is a system for choosing drugs

D.6.1.2 ★ There is a system for drug control, security and maintenance

D.6.1.3 ★ There is a system for emergency drug availability and maintenance

Further Information (see up to date links at **http://quality.resources.machealth.ca**)

College of Physicians & Surgeons of Ontario. Peer Assessment [Internet]. [cited 2010 Jul 22]. Available from: **www.cpso.on.ca/members/peerassessment/default.aspx?id=1944**

Sempowski IP, Brison RJ. Dealing with office emergencies: Stepwise approach for family physicians. CFP [Internet]. 2002 Sept [cited 2010 Jul 22]. Available from: **www.cfp.ca/content/48/9/1464.abstract**

Paediatric emergency equipment and supplies: Guidelines for physician's offices. CFP [Internet]. 2001 Apr [cited 2010 Jul 22];47:797-799. Available from: **www.ncbi.nlm.nih.gov/pmc/articles/PMC2735386/**

Royal Australian College of General Practitioners National Expert Committee on Standards for General Practices. RACGP Standards for General Practices - Criterion 5.2.2 Doctor's bag, Our practice ensures that each GP has access to a doctor's bag; 2007 Jul 18 [cited 2014 Jul 14]. Available from: **www.racgp.org.au/standards/522**

Royal New Zealand College of General Practitioners. Aiming for Excellence – An Assessment Tool for New Zealand General Practice. 3rd ed [monograph online]. New Zealand: Royal New Zealand College of General Practitioners (RNZCGP); 2009. Indicator B.4.6, Practice security is maintained to ensure there is only authorized access to medications and pharmaceutical products; p.41. [cited 2010 Jul 22]. Available from: **www.rnzcgp.org.nz/assets/documents/CORNERSTONE/Aiming-for-Excellence-2009-including-record-review.pdf**

Royal New Zealand College of General Practitioners. Aiming for Excellence – An Assessment Tool for New Zealand General Practice. 3rd ed [monograph online]. New Zealand: Royal New Zealand College of General Practitioners (RNZCGP); 2009. Indicator B.5.1, Medical equipment and resources are available and maintained; p.47. [cited 2010 Jul 22]. Available from: **www.rnzcgp.org.nz/assets/documents/CORNERSTONE/Aiming-for-Excellence-2009-including-record-review.pdf**

College of Physicians & Surgeons of Ontario. Dispensing Drugs [Internet]. 2010 [cited 2014 Jul 14]. Available from: **www.cpso.on.ca/CPSO/media/uploadedfiles/dispensing_drugs.pdf**

Sub-Category D.6 Drugs

Indicator D.6.1
Drugs available in the practice are appropriate, controlled, secure and maintained

Recommended steps for controlling drugs in the practice include authorized access, secure storage, a bi-annual audit, and dispensing records.

Criteria:

D.6.1.1 ★ There is a system for choosing drugs

Interpretation

- The clinical team follows a standard procedure for choosing all drugs to use on and off-site, including in the doctor's bag (e.g., individual or committee members, best-practice guidelines, review schedule, selection of new drugs, review of usage, influence of adverse events on choice of drugs, etc.)

D.6.1.2 ★ There is a system for drug control, security and maintenance

Interpretation

- The practice management can describe:
  - Who is authorized to access controlled, restricted and prescription drugs
  - The secure storage of controlled, restricted and prescription drugs and samples (such as analgesics, narcotics, psychotropic drugs or other potentially dangerous drugs), i.e., they are not kept in the examining rooms
  - Drugs that are in stock and current in the practice
  - The dispensing and/or replacement of drugs including samples
  - How outdated drugs are safely discarded
  - The system that ensures doctors' bags are not accessible to unauthorized people (doctor's bag should be locked in a cupboard or stored in a locked compartment in a vehicle or other clearly non-accessible place when in the office, car or home. There should be a locking device on the bag.)
- The practice management can produce:
  - The results of the bi-annual audit of all drugs
  - A list of controlled, restricted and prescription drugs
  - A record of when narcotics, restricted and prescription drugs have been given to a patient – recorded both in the patient's chart and in a separate record kept with the narcotics container or in the medication cabinet. This record should list the drug, amount dispensed, to whom, by whom and when; it makes internal abuse more difficult, especially in large offices.
  - A regular narcotics count that verifies inventory
- There is a designated person or persons responsible for maintaining the inventory of stock and current drugs that are in the practice and in the doctor's bag

D.6.1.3 ★ There is a system for emergency drug availability and maintenance

Interpretation

- All essential emergency drugs are available in the practice
- There is a designated person or persons responsible for maintaining and keeping current all emergency drugs
- An audit is done following each emergency where drugs were used, to show that the emergency drug use was recorded in the patient's record

Sub-Category D.6 Prescription Management

Indicator D.6.2 Prescription management

Criteria D.6.2.1 ⚖ There is a system for prescription management (which includes organization, security, after-hours, no-visit, pharmacy relationships)

D.6.2.2 ★ There is a system for initial and repeat prescribing without a visit

Further Information (see up to date links at **http://quality.resources.machealth.ca**)

College of Physicians & Surgeons of Ontario. Medical Records [Internet]. 2006 Mar/Apr [cited 2014 Jul 14]. Available from: **www.cpso.on.ca/policies/policies/default.aspx?id=1686**

Ministry of Health and Long-Term Care (Ontario). MedsCheck [Internet]. 2007 [cited 2014 Jul 14]. Available from: **www.health.gov.on.ca/en/public/programs/drugs/medscheck/**

Narcotic Control Regulations, C.R.C., c. 1041. [updated 2010 Jun 28; cited 2010 Jul 21]. Available from: **http://laws.justice.gc.ca/en/C.R.C.-c.1041/FullText.html**

Healthy Environments and Consumer Safety Branch (Health Canada). Information Bulletin for Controlled Substances Licensed Dealers for the Regulations on Benzodiazepines and Other Targeted Substances [Internet]. 2000 Jul 25 [cited 2010 Jul 22].
Benzodiazepines and Other Targeted Substances Regulations, SOR/2000-217. [updated 2010 Jun 28; cited 2010 Jul 22].

This legislation states: "targeted substance" means

(a) a controlled substance that is included in Schedule 1; or

(b) a product or compound that contains a controlled substance that is included in Schedule 1.

Available from: **http://laws-lois.justice.gc.ca/eng/regulations/SOR-2000-217/index.html**

Health Canada. Adverse Reaction Reporting [Internet]. [updated 2010 Jun 10; cited 2010 Jul 22]. Available from: **www.hc-sc.gc.ca/dhp-mps/medeff/report-declaration/index-eng.php**

Ontario College of Pharmacists. Policy on Faxed Prescriptions [Internet]. 2007 May/Jun [cited 2010 Jul 22]. Available from: **www.ocpinfo.com/regulations-standards/policies-guidelines/faxed-prescriptions/**

Winkelaar PG. Lengthy prescription refills. CFP [Internet]. 2002 Sept [cited 2010 Jul 22]. Available from: **www.ncbi.nlm.nih.gov/pubmed/12371302**

Sub-Category D.6 Prescription Management

Indicator D.6.2
Prescription management

Medications ordered for patients are prescribed and managed in the safest manner possible.

Criteria:

D.6.2.1 ⚖ **There is a system for prescription management (which includes organization, security, after-hours, no-visit, pharmacy relationships)**

Interpretation

- The practice management can describe how the clinical team:
  - Provides initial and repeat prescriptions on and off-site, during and outside office hours
  - Reviews prescribed medications in patients taking three or more drugs
  - Identifies and resolves drug-therapy issues
  - Identifies and reports adverse reactions to medications
  - Identifies potential drug interactions
  - Corresponds with pharmacists regarding drug recommendations
  - Documents how drug therapy problems are addressed
  - Limits prescribing to authorized prescribers
  - Uses fax, electronic means and paper for prescribing
- There are no prescription pads left in the examining rooms or where patients can access them; EMR prescription modules cannot be accessed by patients or non-authorized practice team members
- There is an annual prescriptions audit (including initial, repeat and episodic prescriptions and prescriptions made without a visit)

D.6.2.2 ★ **There is a system for initial and repeat prescribing without a visit**

Interpretation

- The practice management can describe how:
  - The clinical team manages prescriptions without a visit (including initial prescriptions and follow-up for repeat prescriptions)
  - Incident reports of improper use of telephone and electronic prescribing are recorded and addressed
  - Medications are reviewed for patients with complex health problems
- An annual patient satisfaction survey includes questions on the process for initial and repeat telephone prescriptions

Sub-Category D.7 Medical Record-keeping

Indicator D.7.1 Medical records are stored or filed safely and securely (see also A.1.1)

Criteria D.7.1.1 ⚖ The content of patients' medical records and related documents (on paper or computer) can be viewed only by authorized individuals

Sub-Category D.7 Medical Record-keeping

Indicator D.7.1
Medical records are stored or filed safely and securely (see also A.1.1)

Steps to ensure that medical records are stored securely and retrievable only by authorized medical staff include safe storage of backup tapes or CDs, computer password protection and lockouts, and an IT strategic plan.

Criteria:

D.7.1.1 ⚖ The content of patients' medical records and related documents (on paper or computer) can be viewed only by authorized individuals

Interpretation

- The content of medical records (paper or computer) are not visible to unauthorized people in the practice's reception area, public places or storage areas
- Records (paper or computer) with identifiable information are not visible to unauthorized people in consulting rooms
- Files that cannot be locked (or are on non-secure computers) are not accessible to unauthorized individuals
- The practice management can describe:
  - The storage and security system for paper patient records and associated documents
  - An overall IT operations plan, storage and security system for electronic medical records and computers that includes:
    - An individual responsible for information technology (IT)
    - A security system of computers and EMRs describing authorization and levels, password protection, screensavers and lockouts
    - A computer backup system for patient data, backup verification, safe storage of backup tapes and CDs
    - External protection including links to other programs, internet access, downloading of material and authorization for loading programs
    - An IT strategic plan, drawn up by the practice, covering three years
- There is an annual audit on safe and secure record-keeping (paper or computer)

Further Information (see up to date links at **http://quality.resources.machealth.ca**)

College of Physicians & Surgeons of Ontario. Medical Records [Internet]. 2006 Mar/Apr [cited 2010 Jul 21]. Available from: **www.cpso.on.ca/policies/policies/default.aspx?id=1686**

Sub-Category D.7 Medical Record-keeping

Indicator D.7.2 Medical records include all essential information necessary to provide quality patient care

Criteria

- **D.7.2.1** ⚖ There is a daily diary of patient appointments
- **D.7.2.2** ⚖ Each patient record meets best practices and CPSO guidelines
- **D.7.2.3** ★ Each patient record has a cumulative patient profile (CPP)
- **D.7.2.4** ★ Telephone conversations are recorded in the medical records
- **D.7.2.5** ★ Notifications to patients of recalls, results, referrals and other contacts are recorded in the medical records
- **D.7.2.6** ★ Clinical management decisions made out-of-office and after-hours are recorded
- **D.7.2.7** ★ There is a biannual audit of patient records

Further Information (see up to date links at **http://quality.resources.machealth.ca**)

College of Physicians & Surgeons of Ontario. Medical Records [Internet]. 2006 Mar/Apr [cited 2010 Jul 21]. Available from: **www.cpso.on.ca/policies/policies/default.aspx?id=1686**

College of Nurses of Ontario. Practice Guideline: Telepractice [Internet]. 2009 [cited 2010 Jul 22]. Available from: **www.cno.org/Global/docs/prac/41041_telephone.pdf**

Smith PC, Araya-Guerra R, Bublitz C, Parnes B, Dickinson LM, Van Vorst R, Westfall JM, Pace WD. Missing Clinical Information During Primary Care Visits. JAMA [Internet]. 2005 Feb 2 [cited 2010 Jul 22];293:565-571. Available from: **http://jama.ama-assn.org/cgi/content/abstract/293/5/565**

Sub-Category D.7 Medical Record-keeping

Indicator D.7.2
Medical records include all essential information necessary to provide quality patient care

Patient records should include cumulative patient profiles, up-to-date lists of problems and medications, telephone conversations, clinical decisions and all other necessary information about the patient and their care in accordance with best-practice guidelines, legal and local standards.

Criteria:

D.7.2.1 ⚖ **There is a daily diary of patient appointments**

Interpretation
- All professional encounters are recorded in the daily diary of appointments
- There is a system to document and follow up on missed appointments

D.7.2.2 ⚖ **Each patient record meets best practices and CPSO guidelines**

Interpretation
- Each patient encounter includes a history, physical examination, provisional diagnosis and treatment plan (including medication decisions)

D.7.2.3 ★ **Each patient record has a cumulative patient profile (CPP)**

Interpretation
- Each patient record has a cumulative and up-to-date list of problems
- Each patient record has a cumulative and up-to-date list of medications
- The chart has a designated place for recording drug allergies and adverse drug reactions

D.7.2.4 ★ **Telephone conversations are recorded in the medical records**

Interpretation
- Each telephone call is managed and clinical plans recorded

D.7.2.5 ★ **Notifications to patients of recalls, results, referrals and other contacts are recorded in the medical records**

Interpretation
- Notification of recalls, results, referrals and other contacts to patients are recorded and signed on the chart

D.7.2.6 ★ **Clinical management decisions made out-of-office and after-hours are recorded**

Interpretation
- Decisions made out of office and after-hours are recorded and communicated

D.7.2.7 ★ **There is a biannual audit of patient records**

Interpretation
- The biannual audit of patient records includes:
  - A random selection of medical records
  - A summary of problems identified and changes made in accordance with the CPSO/regulatory guideline for each practice/provider
  - Assessment of legibility
  - Telephone conversation management and recording
  - Reviews of out-of-office and after-hours records

Sub-Category D.7 Medical Record-keeping

Indicator D.7.3 There is a system to track and manage patients' test results and medical reports

Criteria D.7.3.1 ⚖ The practice team tracks and manages test results, medical reports and investigations and informs patients of the results

D.7.3.2 ⚖ The practice team ensures that all laboratory results and other reports are seen and acted on by the appropriate member of the practice team who requested them or a designated alternate (locum, partner, NP)

Further Information (see up to date links at **http://quality.resources.machealth.ca**)

College of Physicians & Surgeons of Ontario. Medical Records [Internet]. 2006 Mar/Apr [cited 2010 Jul 21]. Available from: **www.cpso.on.ca/policies/policies/default.aspx?id=1686**

White B. Preventing Errors in Your Practice: Four Principles for Better Test-Result Tracking. Fam Pract Manag [Internet]. 2002 Jul/Aug [cited 2010 Jul 22];9(7):41-44. Available from: **www.aafp.org/fpm/20020700/41four.html**

Canadian Medical Protective Association. Responsibility for follow up of investigations [Internet]. 2008 Jun [cited 2014 Jul 14]. Available from: **https://oplfrpd5.cmpa-acpm.ca/-/responsibility-for-follow-up-of-investigations**

MA Coalition for the Prevention of Medical Errors. Communicating Critical Test Results: Safe Practice Recommendations [Internet]. 2003 Mar 17 [cited 2010 Jul 22]. Available from: **www.macoalition.org/documents/CTRPractices.pdf**

Sub-Category D.7 Medical Record-keeping

Indicator D.7.3
There is a system to track and manage patient test results and medical reports

The practice has an effective system in place for managing test results and medical reports, including follow-up of missing results and notification of patients.

Criteria:

D.7.3.1 ⚖ **The practice team tracks and manages patients' test results, medical reports and investigations; follows up on missing results and informs patients of the outcome**

Interpretation

- There is a system for:
  - Tracking and managing patients' test results, medical reports and investigations
  - Notifying patients of test results and reports
  - The follow-up of missing or lost results, including patient responsibility to follow up test results
  - The follow-up of abnormal test results

D.7.3.2 ⚖ **The practice team ensures that all laboratory results and other reports are seen and acted on by the appropriate member of the practice team who requested them or a designated alternate (locum, partner, NP)**

Interpretation

- The practice management can describe:
  - The system used to monitor, review and act on all incoming test results and medical reports
  - How the practice team follows up on missing results and reports
  - How abnormal test results come to the attention of the appropriate provider
- The practice management can identify:
  - The person responsible for acting on incoming test results and reports
  - The designated alternate provider to process test results and medical reports if the primary provider is not present

Sub-Category D.8 Incident Reporting

Indicator D.8.1 There is an incident reporting system to identify and address serious or potentially serious adverse events

Criteria

D.8.1.1 ❊ There is an adverse-incident reporting system

D.8.1.2 ❊ There is a mortality review system

Sub-Category D.8 Incident Reporting

Indicator D.8.1
There is an incident reporting system to identify and address serious or potentially serious adverse events

An incident reporting and management system identifies and addresses adverse events, errors, near-misses, etc.

Criteria:

D.8.1.1 ❋ **There is an adverse-incident reporting system**

Interpretation

- The practice reviews adverse incidents
- The practice summarizes all adverse incidents reported in the past two years, noting follow-up actions taken

D.8.1.2 ❋ **There is a mortality review system**

Interpretation

- The practice management can:
  - Provide a list of all patients who have died in the past two years
  - Describe how each death was reviewed and any follow-up resulting from the review

Further Information (see up to date links at **http://quality.resources.machealth.ca**)

Yaffe MJ, Gupta G, Still S, Boillat M, Russillo B, Schiff B, Sproule D. Morbidity and mortality audits: "How to" for family practice. CFP [Internet]. 2005 Feb [cited 2010 Jul 22].
Available from: **www.ncbi.nlm.nih.gov/pubmed/15751567**

CATEGORY E: EFFECTIVE CLINICAL PRACTICE

Indicators in this category recommend steps for ensuring that patients receive quality clinical care based on best-practice evidence-based guidelines and include the clinical outcomes of lifestyle and prevention, immunization, screening and surveillance, life-cycle clinical management, sexual health, family violence, chronic disease management and palliative care.

The Institute of Medicine defines effective as: "Providing services based on scientific knowledge to all who could benefit, and refraining from providing services to those not likely to benefit (avoiding underuse and overuse, respectively)."

The Ontario Health Quality Council says: "People should receive care that works and is based on the best available scientific information."

Category E has 9 Sub-Categories with 27 Indicators

E.1 Lifestyle and Prevention

Indicator E.1.1 – Smoking cessation

The practice team uses an evidence-based approach to help patients quit smoking, and monitors their progress

Indicator E.1.2 – Alcohol

Recommended ways in which the practice can help patients with alcohol use and abuse problems include screening tools, counselling, medication and referrals to community programs.

Indicator E.1.3 – Diet and exercise

Recommended ways in which the practice can help patients with diet and exercise include a regular assessment of medication, referrals to community resources, and the recording of BMI and waist circumference.

E.2 Immunization

Indicator E.2.1

Baby, childhood and adolescent immunizations

The practice team meets the provincial guidelines for baby, childhood and adolescent immunizations, including providing Public Health with regular updates and reporting adverse reactions.

Indicator E.2.2 – Adult immunizations

The practice team meets the provincial guidelines for adult immunizations, including reporting adverse reactions to Health Canada.

E.3 Surveillance and Screening

Indicator E.3.1 – Screening for colorectal cancer

The practice team meets the provincial guidelines for screening, surveillance and recall for early detection of colorectal cancer.

Indicator E.3.2 – Screening for cervical cancer

The practice team meets the provincial guidelines for screening, surveillance and recall for early detection of cervical cancer.

Indicator E.3.3 – Screening for breast cancer

The practice team meets the provincial guidelines for screening, surveillance and recall for early detection of breast cancer.

E.4 Life Cycle Clinical Management

Indicator E.4.1 – Well baby/child care

The practice team meets the provincial best-practice guidelines for the provision of well baby/child care.

Indicator E.4.2 – Adolescent care

The practice team meets the best-practice guidelines for adolescent care, including sexual health care, immunizations, prescription management, and referrals to Children's Aid.

Indicator E.4.3 – Maternity care

The practice team meets the provincial best-practice guidelines for maternity care, including prenatal screenings and referrals to other care providers.

Indicator E.4.4 – Adult care

The clinical team meets the best-practice guidelines for the care of both men and women.

Indicator E.4.5 – Frail elder care
The clinical team meets the best-practice guidelines for care of the frail elderly, including identifying vulnerable older patients, assessing their cognitive ability, and monitoring medications.

E.5 Sexual Health

Indicator E.5.1 – Sexual health
The provision of sexual health care includes testing and follow-up for HIV/AIDS and STIs, and family planning.

E.6 Family Violence

Indicator E.6.1 – Family violence
The clinical team routinely screens, manages and follows up on victims of family violence.

E.7 Chronic Disease Management

Indicator E.7.1 – Mental health
Best-practice guidelines for the care of patients with mental health disorders include regular medication assessment and shared-care with psychiatrists and other mental health professionals.

Indicator E.7.2 – Diabetes mellitus
Screening and care management for patients with diabetes includes shared-care with specialists and other health professionals and a system for regularly updating patients' records with lab results and other benchmarks.

Indicator E.7.3 – Hypertension
The clinical team meets best-practice guidelines for patients with hypertension, including regular medication assessments.

Indicator E.7.4
Secondary prevention in coronary heart disease (CHD)
The clinical team meets the best-practice guidelines for patients with coronary heart disease (CHD), including regular medication assessments and an annual audit of care.

Indicator E.7.5
Stroke or transient ischemic attacks (TIAs)
Best practice-guidelines for patients with stroke or transient ischemic attacks include a system for care management, regular medication assessments and an annual audit of stroke and TIA patients' records.

Indicator E.7.6 – Asthma
Best-practice guidelines for patients with asthma include a system for care management, regular medication assessments and advice on lifestyle modification.

Indicator E.7.7
Chronic obstructive pulmonary disease (COPD)
Recommended management of patients with chronic obstructive pulmonary disease includes shared-care with specialists, medication assessments and lifestyle modification advice.

Indicator E.7.8 – Hypothyroidism
Recommended management of patients with hypothyroidism includes shared-care with specialists and regular medication assessments.

Indicator E.7.9 – Epilepsy
Recommended management of patients with epilepsy includes shared-care with specialists, regular medication assessments and an annual audit of patients' records.

Indicator E.7.10 – Cancer
Best-practice guidelines for patients with cancer include shared-care with specialists, medication assessments, and carefully maintained records of diagnosis, ongoing treatment and after-care.

E.8 Palliative Care

Indicator E.8.1 – Palliative care
Recommended management of palliative-care patients includes a system of referrals and shared-care and regular medication assessments.

E.9 Open Indicator

Indicator E.9.1 – Open Indicator
This generic indicator allows the practice team to adapt and apply the framework developed for each indicator group to other clinical problems or issues identified as important and relevant to the practice.

Sub-Category E.1 Lifestyle and Prevention

Indicator E.1.1 Smoking cessation

Criteria

E.1.1.1 ★ The practice team has an evidence-based approach to smoking cessation

E.1.1.2 ❃ There is a regular assessment of smoking-cessation medication

E.1.1.3 ❃ The practice team encourages self-care for patients who smoke

Sub-Category E.1 Lifestyle and Prevention

Indicator E.1
Smoking cessation

The practice team uses an evidence-based approach to help patients quit smoking, and monitors their progress

Criteria:

E.1.1.1 ★ The practice team has an evidence-based approach to smoking cessation

Interpretation

- Patients' smoking status and any advice or counselling is recorded on their charts, and warning flags placed on the computer system
- The practice has a list of the smoking status of all patients
- An annual audit monitors the success of the smoking-cessation approach
- A patient satisfaction survey evaluates the smoking-cessation approach

E.1.1.2 ❃ There is a regular assessment of smoking-cessation medication

Interpretation

- The practice management reviews and monitors smoking-cessation prescription and non-prescription medication use

E.1.1.3 ❃ The practice team encourages self-care for patients who smoke

Interpretation

- The practice helps patients find local smoking-cessation programs and access websites, pamphlets, toll-free numbers, etc.

Further information (see up to date links at **http://quality.resources.machealth.ca**)

Center for Addiction and Mental Health. Addiction Toolkit: Smoking Cessation [Internet]. [cited 2015 May 19]. Available from: **www.porticonetwork.ca/web/smoking-toolkit/tools-resources**

Stead LF, Bergson G, Lancaster T. Physician advice for smoking cessation. Cochrane Database of Systematic Reviews [Internet]. 2008 [cited 2015 May 19].
Available from: **http://onlinelibrary.wiley.com/doi/10.1002/14651858.CD000165.pub4/pdf**
Art. No.: CD000165. DOI: 10.1002/14651858.CD000165.pub3

Canadian Cancer Society. Smokers' Helpline [Internet]. [cited 2010 Jul 22].
Available from: **www.smokershelpline.ca/?gclid=CKGxtLiZu6ACFVk65QodZXU1Sg**

Sub-Category E.1 Lifestyle and Prevention

Indicator E.1.2 Alcohol

Criteria

E.1.2.1 ★ The practice team has an evidence-based approach to excess alcohol use

E.1.2.2 ❃ There is a regular medication assessment of alcohol-cessation drugs

E.1.2.3 ❃ The practice team encourages self-care for patients who abuse alcohol

Further Information (see up to date links at **http://quality.resources.machealth.ca**)

Ministry of Health and Long-Term Care (Ontario). Alcohol and Substance Abuse Prevention – The FOCUS Community Program [Internet]. [updated 2009 Jun 16; cited 2014 Jul 14].
Available from: **www.health.gov.on.ca/en/public/publications/hpromo/hpromo.aspx**

Minozzi S, Amato L, Vecchi S, Davoli M. Anticonvulsants for alcohol withdrawal. Cochrane Database of Systematic Reviews [Internet]. 2010 [cited 2010 Jul 22].
Available from: **www.mrw.interscience.wiley.com/cochrane/clsysrev/articles/CD005064/frame.html**
Art. No.: CD005064. DOI: 10.1002/14651858.CD005064.pub3.

Amato L, Minozzi S, Vecchi S, Davoli M. Benzodiazepines for alcohol withdrawal. Cochrane Database of Systematic Reviews [Internet]. 2010 [cited 2010 Jul 22].
Available from: **www.mrw.interscience.wiley.com/cochrane/clsysrev/articles/CD005063/frame.html**
Art. No.: CD005063. DOI: 10.1002/14651858.CD005063.pub3.

Scottish Intercollegiate Guidelines Network. The management of harmful drinking and alcohol dependence in primary care: A national clinical guideline [Internet]. 2003 Sept [cited 2010 Jul 22].
Available from: **www.sign.ac.uk/pdf/sign74.pdf**

Alcoholics Anonymous. The A.A. Preamble [Internet]. [cited 2015 May 19].
Available from: **www.aa.org/assets/en_US/aa-literature/smf-92-aa-preamble**

Sub-Category E.1 Lifestyle and Prevention

Indicator E.1.2
Alcohol

Recommended ways in which the practice can help patients with alcohol use and abuse problems include screening tools, counselling, medication and referrals to community programs.

Criteria:

E.1.2.1 ★ The practice team has an evidence-based approach to excess alcohol use

Interpretation

- There is an evidence-based approach for patients who use/abuse alcohol including tools such as warning flags, screening, and brief or extensive advice and counselling; such assistance is recorded on the chart
- The practice management can produce:
  - An updated list of all patients who use alcohol to excess
  - An annual audit that monitors the success of the alcohol-reduction approach
  - A patient satisfaction survey that evaluates the alcohol-reduction approach

E.1.2.2 ✻ There is a regular medication assessment of alcohol-cessation drugs

Interpretation

- The practice reviews and monitors alcohol withdrawal and cessation prescription medication

E.1.2.3 ✻ The practice team encourages self-care for patients who abuse alcohol

Interpretation

- Patients are referred to local alcohol reduction programs and told how to access websites, pamphlets, toll-free numbers, etc.
- Information on alcohol reduction is provided to patients

Sub-Category E.1 Lifestyle and Prevention

Indicator E.1.3 Diet and exercise

Criteria	**E.1.3.1**	★	The practice team uses an evidence-based approach to diet and exercise
	E.1.3.2	❋	There is a regular medication assessment of drugs for weight reduction
	E.1.3.3	❋	The practice encourages diet and exercise self-care

Sub-Category E.1 Lifestyle and Prevention

Indicator E.1.3
Diet and exercise

Recommended ways in which the practice can help patients with diet and exercise include a regular assessment of medication, referrals to community resources, and the recording of BMI and waist circumference.

Criteria:

E.1.3.1 ★ The practice team uses an evidence-based approach to diet and exercise

Interpretation

- There is an evidence-based approach for recommending diet and exercise: regular physical activity and advice is recorded on the chart as well as BMI and waist circumference
- There is an updated list of all patients who have an elevated or reduced BMI or waist circumference

E.1.3.2 ✻ There is a regular assessment of medication for weight reduction

Interpretation

- The practice management reviews and monitors weight-reduction and eating-disorder medication use

E.1.3.3 ✻ The practice team encourages diet and exercise self-care

Interpretation

- Patients are referred to local dietitians and diet and exercise programs and told how to access websites, pamphlets, toll-free numbers, etc.

Further Information (see up to date links at **http://quality.resources.machealth.ca**)

Shaw KA, Gennat HC, O'Rourke P, Del Mar C. Exercise for overweight or obesity. Cochrane Database of Systematic Reviews [Internet]. 2006 [cited 2010 Jul 22].
Available from: **www.mrw.interscience.wiley.com/cochrane/clsysrev/articles/CD003817/frame.html**
Art. No.: CD003817. DOI: 10.1002/14651858.CD003817.pub3.

Padwal RS, Rucker D, Li SK, Curioni C, Lau DCW. Long-term pharmacotherapy for obesity and overweight. Cochrane Database of Systematic Reviews [Internet]. 2003 [cited 2010 Jul 22].
Available from: **www.mrw.interscience.wiley.com/cochrane/clsysrev/articles/CD004094/frame.html**
Art. No.: CD004094. DOI: 10.1002/14651858.CD004094.pub2.

Stanford School of Medicine. Stanford Self-Management Programs [Internet]. [cited 2010 Jul 22].
Available from: **http://patienteducation.stanford.edu/programs/**

Lau D.C.W., Douketis J.D., Morrison K.M., Hramiak I.M., Sharma A.M., Ur E., for members of the Obesity Canada Clinical Practice Guidelines Expert Panel. 2006 Canadian clinical practice guidelines on the management and prevention of obesity in adults and children [summary]. [Internet]. 2007[cited 15 Nov 2010]. CMAJ 2007; 176 (8). doi:10.1503/cmaj.061409. Available from: **www.cmaj.ca/cgi/data/176/8/S1/DC1/1**

Sub-Category E.2 Immunization

Indicator E.2.1 Baby, childhood and adolescent immunizations

Criteria

E.2.1.1 ★ The practice team meets provincial guidelines for baby, childhood and adolescent immunizations

E.2.1.2 ★ The clinical team reports adverse reactions to immunizations

Sub-Category E.2 Immunization

Indicator E.2.1
Baby, childhood and adolescent immunizations

The practice team meets the provincial guidelines for baby, childhood and adolescent immunizations, including providing Public Health with regular updates and reporting adverse reactions.

Criteria:

E.2.1.1 ★ The practice team meets provincial guidelines for baby, childhood and adolescent immunizations

Interpretation

- The practice has a system for immunizing babies, children and adolescents
- The practice provides Public Health with regular updates on baby, childhood and adolescent vaccinations
- The practice management can produce:
  - A baby, childhood and adolescent immunization surveillance and recall list
  - The percentage of children who have received required full immunization by 7 years
  - The percentage of children who have received required full immunization by 14-16 years
  - The percentage of girls and women who have been offered, and received or rejected, HPV vaccination

E.2.1.2 ★ The clinical team reports adverse reactions to immunizations

Interpretation

- There is a system for recording all adverse reactions to immunizations and reporting them to Health Canada

Further Information (see up to date links at **http://quality.resources.machealth.ca**)

Public Health Agency of Canada. Canada Immunization Guide. [cited 2015 Oct. 08].
Available from: **www.phac-aspc.gc.ca/publicat/cig-gci/index-eng.php**

Niagara Regional. Infectious Diseases & Vaccinations [Internet]. 2010 [cited 2010 Jul 22].
Available from: **www.regional.niagara.on.ca/living/health_wellness/disease-prevent/default.aspx**

Ontario's immunization schedule. [cited 2015 Oct 08].
Available from: **www.health.gov.on.ca/en/public/programs/immunization/static/immunization_tool.html**

Ministry of Health & Long-Term Care (Ontario). Immunization: Fact Sheets and Patient Tools [Internet]. 2003 [updated 2014 Feb 07; cited 2014 Jul 14].
Available from: **www.health.gov.on.ca/en/pro/programs/immunization/resources.aspx**

Ministry of Health & Long-Term Care (Ontario). Immunization Provider Information Package [Internet]. 2002 [updated 2009 Jun 12; cited 2010 Jul 22].
Available from: **www.health.gov.on.ca/english/providers/program/immun/provinfo_pack.html**

Health Canada. MedEffectTM Canada - Adverse Reaction Database and On-line reporting [Internet]. [updated 2010 Jun 28; cited 2010 Jul 22]. Available from: **www.hc-sc.gc.ca/dhp-mps/medeff/databasdon/index-eng.php**

Sub-Category E.2 Immunization

Indicator E.2.2 Adult immunizations

Criteria

E.2.1.1 ★ The practice team meets provincial guidelines for adult immunizations

E.2.1.2 ★ The clinical team reports adverse reactions to adult immunizations

Sub-Category E.2 Immunization

Indicator E.2.2
Adult immunizations

The practice team meets the provincial guidelines for adult immunizations, including reporting adverse reactions to Health Canada

Criteria:

E.2.1.1 ★ The practice team meets provincial guidelines for adult immunization

Interpretation

- The practice management can describe:
  - Its system for reviewing immunization procedures against new provincial guidelines
  - Its system of offering immunization to those women who require it prior to pregnancy
- The practice management can produce:
  - An adult immunization surveillance and recall list
  - The percentage of adults who are up to date in adult immunizations
  - The percentage of adults aged 65 or older who have been offered, and received or refused, influenza vaccine and pneumococcal vaccine
  - The percentage of rubella-immune women of childbearing age

E.2.1.2 ★ The clinical team reports adverse reactions to immunizations

Interpretation

- There is a system for recording all adverse reactions to immunizations and reporting them to Health Canada

Further Information (see up to date links at **http://quality.resources.machealth.ca**)

Ontario's immunization schedule. [cited 2015 Oct 08].
Available from: **www.health.gov.on.ca/en/public/programs/immunization/static/immunization_tool.html**

Center for Disease Control and Prevention (US) Recommended Adult Immunization Schedule – United States, 2014 [Internet]. 2014 [cited 2014 Jul 14].
Available from: **www.aafp.org/dam/AAFP/documents/patient_care/immunizations/adult-immunization-schedule.pdf**

Public Health Agency of Canada. Human Papilloma Virus (HPV) Prevention and HPV Vaccine: Questions and Answers [Internet]. [updated 2007 Jun 18; 2010 Jul 22].
Available from: **www.phac-aspc.gc.ca/std-mts/hpv-vph/hpv-vph-vaccine-eng.php**

Public Health Agency of Canada. Canadian Immunization Guide. 7th ed [monograph online]. Ottawa: Public Health Agency of Canada; 2006. Part 4 Active Immunizing Agents, Pneumococcal Vaccine. [cited 2010 Jul 22].
Available from: **www.phac-aspc.gc.ca/publicat/cig-gci/p04-pneu-eng.php**

Merck Frosst Canada Ltd. Consumer Information - Pneumovax® 23 [Internet]. [updated 2009 Jul 15; cited 2010 Jul 22]. Available from: **www.merck.ca/assets/en/pdf/products/ci/PNEUMOVAX_23-CI_E.pdf**

Sub-Category E.3 Surveillance and Screening

Indicator E.3.1 Screening for colorectal cancer

Criteria

E.3.1.1 ★ **ColonCancerCheck program:** The practice team can report the percentage of eligible patients aged 50 to 74 who are in the program

E.3.1.2 ★ **Screening rate:** The practice team can report the percentage of eligible patients aged 50-74 who have had an FOBT in the preceding two years

E.3.1.3 ★ **Time to referral:** The practice team can report the percentage of patients with positive FOBT results who are notified and have follow-up to a colonoscopy within two weeks

E.3.1.4 ★ **Family history:** The practice team has a list of patients with a family history of colorectal cancer

E.3.1.5 ★ **Over-screening rate:** The practice can report the percentage of patients aged 50-74 with more than one FOBT in the preceding two years

Further Information (see up to date links at **http://quality.resources.machealth.ca**)

Ministry of Health & Long-Term Care. ColonCancerCheck [Internet]. 2008 [updated 2010 Apr 12; cited 2010 Jul 22]. Available from: **http://coloncancercheck.ca/**

Sub-Category E.3 Surveillance and Screening

Indicator E.3.1
Screening for colorectal cancer

The practice team meets the provincial guidelines for screening, surveillance and recall for early detection of colorectal cancer.

Criteria:

E.3.1.1 ★ ColonCancerCheck program: The practice team can report the percentage of eligible patients aged 50 to 74 who are in the program

Interpretation

- The practice has a system for screening, surveillance and recall of all eligible patients for FOBT (including family history)
- There is a list of all eligible patients linked to the ColonCancerCheck program

E.3.1.2 ★ Screening rate: The practice team can report the percentage of eligible patients aged 50-74 who have had an FOBT in the preceding two years

Interpretation

- The practice management can produce:
  - A report on the percentage of eligible patients who have had an FOBT
  - The results of an annual screening audit and a plan to improve the results

E.3.1.3 ★ Time to referral: The practice team can report the percentage of patients with positive FOBT results who are notified and have follow-up to a colonoscopy within two weeks

Interpretation

- The practice has a system for follow-up of all FOBT results
- The clinical team informs patients of their FOBT results
- The practice can report the percentage of eligible patients aged 50-74 with a positive FOBT who receive notification of results and follow-up to a colonoscopy within two weeks

E.3.1.4 ★ Family history: The practice team has a list of patients with a family history of colorectal cancer

Interpretation

- The practice management can produce a list of patients with a first-degree family history of colorectal cancer

E.3.1.5 ★ Over-screening rate: The practice team can report the percentage of patients aged 50-74 with more than one FOBT in the preceding two years

Interpretation

- There is a list of patients who have had more than one FOBT in the preceding year and there is a plan in place to reduce their number

Sub-Category E.3 Surveillance and Screening

Indicator E.3.2 Screening for cervical cancer

Criteria

E.3.2.1 ★ **Screening rate:** The practice team can report the percentage of eligible women up to age 70 who have had a pap test in the preceding three years

E.3.2.2 ★ **Time to referral:** The practice team can report the percentage of women with abnormal pap test results who receive notification and appropriate follow-up within two weeks

E.3.2.3 ★ **Over-screening rate:** The practice team can report the percentage of eligible women up to age 70 who have had more than one normal pap test in the preceding two to three years

Further Information (see up to date links at **http://quality.resources.machealth.ca**)

Ontario Cervical Screening Program (Cancer Care Ontario). Ontario Cervical Screening Practice Guidelines [Internet]. 2005 Jun [cited 2010 Jul 22].
Available from: **www.cancercare.on.ca/common/pages/UserFile.aspx?fileId=13104**

Cancer Care Ontario. About the Ontario Cervical Screening Program [Internet]. [updated 2009 Nov 23; cited 2010 Jul 22].
Available from: **www.cancercare.on.ca/pcs/screening/cervscreening/OCSP/**

Cervical Screening Guidelines Development Committee of the Ontario Cervical Screening Program and the Gynecology Cancer Disease Site Group of Cancer Care Ontario. Cervical Screening: Guideline Recommendations [Internet]. 2011 Oct 5 [cited 2015 May 19].
Available from: **https://www.cancercare.on.ca/common/pages/UserFile.aspx?fileId=124511**

Sub-Category E.3 Surveillance and Screening

Indicator E.3.2
Screening for cervical cancer

The practice team meets the provincial guidelines for screening, surveillance and recall for early detection of cervical cancer.

Criteria:

E.3.2.1 ★ Screening rate: The practice team can report the percentage of eligible women up to age 70 who have had a pap test in the preceding three years

Interpretation

- There is a system for screening, surveillance and recall of all eligible women for cervical pap smears (cervical cytology screening should be initiated within three years of first vaginal sexual activity, i.e., vaginal intercourse, vaginal/oral and/or vaginal/digital sexual activity)
- The practice management can report:
  - The percentage of eligible women who have had pap smears in the past three years
  - The results of an annual screening audit and a plan to improve the results

E.3.2.2 ★ Time to referral: The practice team can report the percentage of women with abnormal pap test results who receive notification and appropriate follow-up within two weeks

Interpretation

- There is a system for follow-up of all pap smear results
- The practice informs women of the results of their pap smears
- The practice can report the percentage of women with abnormal pap smears who received notification of results and follow-up, including referral, within two weeks

E.3.2.3 ★ Over-screening rate: The practice team can report the percentage of eligible women to age 70 who have had more than one normal pap test in the preceding two to three years

Interpretation

- There is a list of women who have had more than one normal pap test in the preceding two to three years and a plan in place to reduce their number (this does not apply to women with previous abnormal pap smears)

Sub-Category E.3 Surveillance and Screening

Indicator E.3.3 Screening for breast cancer

Criteria

E.3.3.1 ★ **Ontario Breast Screening Program:** The practice team can report the percentage of eligible women aged 50-74 who are in the program

E.3.3.2 ★ **Screening rate:** The practice team can report the percentage of eligible women aged 50-74 who have had a mammogram in the preceding two years

E.3.3.3 ★ **Time to referral:** The practice team can report the percentage of women with abnormal mammogram results who receive notification and appropriate follow-up within two weeks

E.3.3.4 ★ **Family history:** The practice team has a list of women patients with a family history of breast cancer in a first-degree relative

E.3.3.5 ★ **Over-screening rate:** The practice team can report the percentage of eligible women aged 50-74 with more than one normal mammogram in the preceding two years

Further Information (see up to date links at **http://quality.resources.machealth.ca**)

Cancer Care Ontario. The Ontario Breast Screening Program [Internet]. [updated 2009 Dec 29; cited 2010 Jul 22]. Available from: **www.cancercare.on.ca/pcs/screening/breastscreening/OBSP/**

Cancer Care Ontario. OBSP Screening Site Locations [Internet]. [updated 2009 Dec 29; cited 2010 Jul 22]. Available from: **www.cancercare.on.ca/pcs/screening/breastscreening/locations/**

Sub-Category E.3 Surveillance and Screening

Indicator E.3.3
Screening for breast cancer

The practice team meets the provincial guidelines for screening, surveillance and recall for early detection of breast cancer.

Criteria:

E.3.3.1 ★ Ontario Breast Screening Program: The practice team can report the percentage of eligible women aged 50-74 who are in the program

Interpretation

- The practice has a system for breast-cancer screening, surveillance and recall for all eligible women (including family history)
- The practice can produce a list of all eligible women linked to the Ontario Breast Screening Program

E.3.3.2 ★ Screening rate: The practice team can report the percentage of eligible women aged 50-74 who have had a mammogram in the preceding two years

Interpretation

- The practice can produce:
  - The percentage of eligible women who have had a mammogram
  - The results of an annual screening audit and a plan to improve the results

E.3.3.3 ★ Time to referral: The practice team can report the percentage of women with abnormal mammogram results who receive notification and appropriate follow-up within two weeks

Interpretation

- The practice has a system for follow-up of all mammogram results
- The practice informs all eligible women of their mammogram results
- The practice can report the percentage of eligible women aged 50-74 with a positive mammogram who are notified of results and follow-up/referral

E.3.3.4 ★ Family History: The practice team has a list of women patients with a family history of breast cancer in a first-degree relative

Interpretation

- The practice can produce a list of all women with a first-degree family history of breast cancer

E.3.3.5 ★ Over-screening rate: The practice team can report the percentage of eligible women aged 50-74 with more than one normal mammogram in the preceding two years

Interpretation

- There is a list of women who have had more than one mammogram in the preceding two years and there is a plan in place to reduce their number

Sub-Category E.4 Life Cycle Clinical Management

Indicator E.4.1 Well baby/child care

Criteria

E.4.1.1 ★ Well-baby/child visits are based on best-practice guidelines

E.4.1.2 ⚖ The clinical team refers appropriately to Children's Aid

E.4.1.3 ★ The practice team encourages access to parenting, well baby/child self-care programs and resources

Further Information (see up to date links at **http://quality.resources.machealth.ca**)

College of Family Physicians of Canada. Rourke Baby Record [Internet]. 2010 [updated 2010 Mar 9; cited 2010 Jul 22]. Available from: **www.cfpc.ca/projectassets/templates/resource.aspx?id=1126&langType=4105**

Limbos MM, Joyce DP, Roberts GJ. Nipissing District Developmental Screen: Patterns of use by physicians in Ontario. Can Fam Physician [Internet]. 2010 Feb [cited 2010 Jul 22];56(2):e66-e72. Available from: **www.cfp.ca/cgi/content/abstract/56/2/e66**

Ministry of Child and Youth Services (Ontario). Reporting child abuse and neglect [Internet]. 2010 [updated 2010 Apr 27; cited 2010 Jul 22]. Available from: **www.children.gov.on.ca/htdocs/English/topics/childrensaid/reportingabuse/index.aspx**

Ontario Association of Children's Aid Societies. Locate a Society [Internet]. 2015 [cited 2015 Oct 08] Available from: **www.oacas.org/childrens-aid/locate-a-childrens-aid-society/**

College of Physicians & Surgeons of Ontario. Mandatory Reporting: Contact Information for making Mandatory Reports [Internet]. 2006 May [cited 2010 Jul 22]. Available from: **www.cpso.on.ca/uploadedFiles/downloads/cpsodocuments/policies/policies/MandRepCONTACTinfo.pdf**

Sub-Category E.4 Life Cycle Clinical Management

Indicator E.4.1
Well baby/child care

The practice team meets the provincial best-practice guidelines for the provision of well baby/child care. (See also E.2 Immunization and A.3 Mandatory Reporting.)

Criteria:

E.4.1.1 ★ Well-baby/child visits are based on best-practice guidelines

Interpretation

- The practice has a system for well baby/child surveillance, screening and recall
- The practice uses evidence-based best practices (e.g., as outlined in the Rourke Baby Record and the Nipissing District Developmental Screen)
- There is an annual audit of well baby/child care and a plan to improve the results

E.4.1.2 ⚖ The clinical team refers appropriately to Children's Aid

Interpretation

- Clinical team members have access to information on and understand their obligations regarding child abuse and neglect under Ontario's Child and Family Services Act (the duty to report applies to any child who is, or appears to be, under the age of 16 years, as well as children subject to a child protection order who are 16 and 17 years old)
- There is a designated contact person for child protection in the practice
- There is a record of clinical team training in child protection, updated every three years

E.4.1.3 ★ The practice team encourages access to parenting, well baby/child self-care programs and resources

Interpretation

- The practice team helps parents find local community programs such as Healthy Babies/Healthy Children, and access websites, pamphlets, toll-free numbers, etc.

Sub-Category E.4 Life Cycle Clinical Management

Indicator E.4.2 Adolescent care

Criteria **E.4.2.1** ★ Adolescent care is based on best-practice guidelines

E.4.1.3 ★ The practice team encourages access to self-care programs and resources

Sub-Category E.4 Life Cycle Clinical Management

Indicator E.4.2
Adolescent care

The practice team meets the best-practice guidelines for provision of adolescent care, including sexual health care, immunizations, prescription management, and referrals to Children's Aid.

Criteria:

E.4.2.1 ★ Adolescent care is based on best-practice guidelines

Interpretation

- There is a system for adolescent patient surveillance, screening and recall
- The practice team promotes best practices for adolescents (i.e., lifestyle, sexual health, immunization)
- The practice conducts an annual audit of a random sample of adolescent patient records (including lifestyle, immunization, surveillance and screening, and drugs) and has a plan to improve the results.

E.4.2.2 ★ The practice team encourages access to self-care programs and resources

Interpretation

- The practice management helps adolescents find local community programs and access websites, pamphlets, toll-free numbers, etc.

Further Information (see up to date links at **http://quality.resources.machealth.ca**)

A variety of reviews of best practices for adolescents can be viewed at the Cochrane reviews:
The Cochrane Collaboration. Cochrane Reviews [Internet]. 2010 [cited 2010 Jul 22].
Available from: **www.cochrane.org/cochrane-reviews**

Stanford School of Medicine. Stanford Self-Management Programs [Internet]. [cited 2010 Jul 22].
Available from: **http://patienteducation.stanford.edu/programs/**

Sub-Category E.4 Life Cycle Clinical Management

Indicator E.4.3 Maternity care

Criteria	**E.4.3.1**	★	Antenatal care is based on provincial best-practice guidelines
	E.4.3.2	❃	The practice team promotes access to self-care programs and resources

Sub-Category E.4 Life Cycle Clinical Management

Indicator E.4.3
Maternity care

The practice team meets the provincial best-practice guidelines for maternity care, including prenatal screenings and referrals to other care providers.

Criteria:

E.4.3.1 ★ Antenatal care is based on provincial best-practice guidelines (see also G.1.1.2 Integrated and Continuous – Shared-care with specialists in obstetrics, psychiatry and chronic disease management)

Interpretation

- The practice has a system for providing antenatal care
- First antenatal appointments are provided early enough to meet IPS screening requirements (Integrated Prenatal Screening at nine weeks)
- There is a system for referring pregnant patients to other care providers that includes written materials for patients on choosing an obstetrician, family physician or midwife (the clinical team works with them for full care or shared-care) and other referrals related to pregnancy
- The practice undertakes an annual audit of antenatal care and has a plan to improve the results

E.4.3.2 ❃ The practice team promotes access to self-care programs and resources

Interpretation

- The practice helps patients find community resources and prenatal programs as well as websites, pamphlets, toll-free numbers, etc.

Further Information (see up to date links at **http://quality.resources.machealth.ca**)

Ontario Medical Association & Ministry of Health & Long-Term Care (Ontario). Antenatal Record Form 1 & 2 [Internet]. 2008 [updated 2014 Aug 14; cited 2014 Jul 14].
Available from: **www.forms.ssb.gov.on.ca/mbs/ssb/forms/ssbforms.nsf/QuickResults?Openform&ENV=WWE&SRCH=1&MIN=&BRN=&PRG=&TIT=antenatal+record+2&NO=&SRT=T&NEW=&STR=1&MAX=10**

Government of Canada. Having a Baby [Internet]. [updated 2014 May 22; cited 2014 Jul 14].
Available from: **www.servicecanada.gc.ca/eng/lifeevents/baby.shtml**

Stanford School of Medicine. Stanford Self-Management Programs [Internet]. [cited 2010 Jul 22].
Available from: **http://patienteducation.stanford.edu/programs/**

Sub-Category E.4 Life Cycle Clinical Management

Indicator E.4.4 Adult care

Criteria **E.4.4.1** ★ Adult care is based on best-practice guidelines

E.4.4.2 ❃ The practice team encourages access to self-care programs and resources

Sub-Category E.4 Life Cycle Clinical Management

Indicator E.4.4
Adult care

The clinical team meets the best-practice guidelines for care of both men and women. (See also E.1 Lifestyle and Prevention, E.2 Immunization, E.3 Surveillance and Screening, and D.6 Drugs.)

Criteria:

E.4.4.1 ★ Adult care is based on best-practice guidelines

Interpretation

- The practice management has a system for providing adult care that includes lifestyle issues, immunization, surveillance and screening, and prescription management; and which differs for women and men (e.g., menopause management, prostate health, etc.)
- There is a system to provide follow-up care for identified problems
- The practice undertakes an annual audit of a random sample of adult patients' records (including record review, surveillance and screening, a problem list, and a cumulative patient profile that includes lifestyle, immunizations, allergies, medications and family history) and has a plan to improve the results

E.4.4.2 ✻ The practice team encourages access to self-care programs and resources

Interpretation

- The practice helps adult patients find local community programs, websites, pamphlets, toll-free numbers, etc.

Further Information (see up to date links at **http://quality.resources.machealth.ca**)

College of Physicians & Surgeons of Ontario. Medical Records [Internet]. 2006 Mar/Apr [cited 2010 Jul 21]. Available from: **www.cpso.on.ca/policies/policies/default.aspx?id=1686**

Society of Obstetricians and Gynaecologists of Canada. Women's Health Information – Menopause [Internet]. [cited 2014 Jul 14]. Available from: **http://sogc.org/publications/menopause/**

American Cancer Society. Prostate Cancer: Early Detection [Internet]. [cited 2010 Jul 22]. Available from: **www.cancer.org/docroot/CRI/content/CRI_2_6x_Prostate_Cancer_Early_Detection.asp?sitearea=&level**

Stanford School of Medicine. Stanford Self-Management Programs [Internet]. [cited 2010 Jul 22]. Available from: **http://patienteducation.stanford.edu/programs/**

Sub-Category E.4 Life Cycle Clinical Management

Indicator E.4.5 Frail elder care

Criteria

E.4.5.1 ★ Frail elder care is based on best-practice guidelines

E.4.5.2 ❃ Dementia/cognitive impairment care is based on best-practice guidelines

E.4.5.3 ❃ The practice team encourages access to self-care programs and resources

Further Information (see up to date links at **http://quality.resources.machealth.ca**)

Guidelines and Protocols Advisory Committee (BC). Frailty in Older Adults - Early Identification and Management [Internet]. 2008 Oct 1 [cited 2014 Jul 08].
Available from: **www.bcguidelines.ca/guideline_frailty.html**

Stanford School of Medicine. Stanford Self-Management Programs [Internet]. [cited 2010 Jul 22].
Available from: **http://patienteducation.stanford.edu/programs/**

Guidelines and Protocols Advisory Committee (BC). Cognitive Impairment in the Elderly – Recognition, Diagnosis and Management [Internet]. 2007 Jul 15 [cited 2015 Oct 08] Available from: **http://www2.gov.bc.ca/gov/content/health/practitioner-professional-resources/bc-guidelines/cognitive-impairment**

Lindsay P, Bayley M, Hellings C, Hill M, Woodbury E, Phillips S. Selected topics in stroke management. Vascular cognitive impairment and dementia. In: Canadian best practice recommendations for stroke care. CMAJ [Internet]. 2008 Dec 2 [cited 2010 Jul 22];179(12 Suppl):E67-70.
Available from: **www.strokebestpractices.ca/index.php/cognition-mood/vascular-cognitive-impairment-and-dementia/**

Sub-Category E.4 Life Cycle Clinical Management

Indicator E.4.5
Frail elder care

The clinical team meets the best-practice guidelines for care of the frail elderly, including identifying vulnerable older patients, assessing their cognitive ability, and monitoring medications. (See also E.2.2 Adult Immunizations.)

Criteria:

E.4.5.1 ★ Frail elder care is based on best-practice guidelines

Interpretation

- The practice has a system for identifying vulnerable older patients (including those who were, or are, hospitalized; on poly-pharmacy; less mobile; or at risk of falls)
- The clinical team routinely assesses the driving safety of vulnerable older adults
- The practice undertakes an annual audit of a sample of vulnerable older patients' records (including frail older patients who were/are hospitalized, on poly-pharmacy, or at risk of falls) and has a plan to improve the results
- The practice management maintains a list of vulnerable older patients

E.4.5.2 ❄ Dementia/cognitive impairment care is based on best-practice guidelines

Interpretation

- The clinical team:
  - Assesses, reviews and documents cognitive ability and functional status if a vulnerable older patient is new to the practice or is admitted to or discharged from hospital
  - Reviews and monitors medications if a patient has symptoms of cognitive impairment
  - Offers patients with dementia and their caregivers education about safety, dealing with conflicts at home, and caregiver support
- The practice undertakes an annual audit of a sample of patients' records with cognitive impairment and has a plan to improve the results

E.4.5.3 ❄ The practice team encourages access to self-care programs and resources

Interpretation

- The practice helps patients find local community programs, websites, pamphlets, toll-free numbers, etc.

Sub-Category E.5 Sexual Health

Indicator E.5.1 Sexual health

Criteria

E.5.1.1 ★ Sexual health care is based on best-practice guidelines

E.5.1.2 ❋ The practice team encourages access to self-care programs and resources

Sub-Category E.5 Sexual Health

Indicator E.5.1
Sexual health

The provision of sexual health care includes testing and follow-up for HIV/AIDS and STIs, and family planning.

Criteria:

E.5.1.1 ★ Sexual health care is based on best-practice guidelines

Interpretation

- The practice:
  - Has a system for the provision of sexual health services including family planning, contraception, emergency contraception, preconception counselling and access to terminations (See also E.2.2 Adult Immunizations)
  - Provides care for sexually transmitted infections, including prevention, investigation, management, follow-up, contacts, reporting and referral
  - Conducts an annual audit of a sample of records of patients with STIs and has a plan to improve the results
  - Provides pre- and post-test counselling, testing and follow-up for patients requiring HIV/AIDS testing
  - Conducts an annual audit of a sample of records of patients who have had HIV/AIDS tests in the past two years

E.5.1.2 ❋ The practice team encourages access to self-care programs and resources

Interpretation

- The practice helps patients find local community programs, websites, pamphlets, toll-free numbers, etc.

Further Information (see up to date links at **http://quality.resources.machealth.ca**)

Canadian Federation for Sexual Health. Home [Internet]. [cited 2010 Jul 22]. Available from: **www.cfsh.ca/**

Public Health Agency of Canada. HIV-AIDS Guidelines [Internet]. [updated 2006 Jul 19; cited 2010 Jul 22]. Available from: **www.phac-aspc.gc.ca/aids-sida/guide/index-eng.php**

College of Physicians & Surgeons of Ontario. The Practice Guide: Medical Professionalism and College Policies [Internet]. 2007 [cited 2010 Jul 22]. Available from: **www.cpso.on.ca/uploadedFiles/policies/guides/PracticeGuideExtract_08.pdf**

Sub-Category E.6 Family Violence

Indicator E.6.1 Family violence

Criteria **E.6.1.1** ❋ The clinical team routinely screens, manages and follows up on patients identified as victims of family violence

E.6.1.2 ❋ The practice team promotes access to self-care programs and resources

Sub-Category E.6 Family Violence

Indicator E.6.1
Family violence

The clinical team routinely screens, manages and follows up on victims of family violence.

Criteria:

E.6.1.1 ❃ **The clinical team routinely screens, manages and follows up on patients identified as victims of family violence**

Interpretation

- The clinical team screens all females over the age of 14 (routine screening means that all women over 14 are asked verbally about domestic abuse whether or not symptoms or signs are present and whether or not the provider suspects abuse has occurred)
- The clinical team ensures that screening will be non-judgmental, culturally competent, confidential and safe (e.g., education, CPD activities)

E.6.1.2 ❃ **The practice team promotes access to self-care programs and resources**

Interpretation

- The practice team helps patients find safe shelters, local community programs, websites, pamphlets, toll-free numbers, etc.

Further Information (see up to date links at **http://quality.resources.machealth.ca**)

Public Health Agency of Canada: Stop Family Violence. [cited 2015 Oct 08]. Available from: **www.phac-aspc.gc.ca/sfv-avf/index-eng.php**

Housing Help Centre. Find a Women's Shelter [Internet]. 2009 [cited 2010 Jul 22]. Available from: **www.housinghelpcentre.org/shelterslisting**

Stanford School of Medicine. Stanford Self-Management Programs [Internet]. [cited 2010 Jul 22]. Available from: **http://patienteducation.stanford.edu/programs/**

Sub-Category E.7 Chronic Disease Management

Indicator E.7.1 Mental health

Criteria

E.7.1.1 ★ Mental health care is based on best-practice guidelines

E.7.1.2 ❃ There is a regular medication assessment for patients with mental health disorders

E.7.1.3 ❃ The practice team promotes access to self-care programs and resources

Sub-Category E.7 Chronic Disease Management

Indicator E.7.1
Mental health

Best-practice guidelines for the care of patients with mental health disorders include regular medication assessment and shared-care with psychiatrists and other mental health professionals.

Criteria:

E.7.1.1 ★ Mental health care is based on best-practice guidelines

Interpretation

- The practice has a system for managing patients with mental health disorders, including referral practices and shared-care with psychiatrists and other mental health professionals (see G.1.1 Continuity of Care)
- The practice maintains a list of patients with mental health disorders that also identifies those who have agreed to regular follow-up
- The practice conducts an annual audit of a sample of mental health patients' records and has a plan to improve the results

E.7.1.2 ❃ There is a regular medication assessment for patients with mental health disorders

Interpretation

- The practice has a system to monitor patients with mental disorders, including sub-optimal response, adverse effects and routine lab tests; and conducts regular medication assessments. There is a plan to resolve any problems identified (See also D.6.2 Prescription Management)

E.7.1.3 ❃ The practice team promotes access to self-care programs and resources

Interpretation

- The practice helps patients with mental health disorders find local community programs, websites, pamphlets, toll-free numbers, self-care, etc.

Further Information (see up to date links at **http://quality.resources.machealth.ca**)

Mood Disorders Association of Ontario. Links [Internet]. 2009 [cited 2010 Jul 22]. Available from: **www.mooddisorders.ca/links**

Burgess SSA, Geddes J, Hawton KKE, Taylor MJ, Townsend E, Jamison K, Goodwin G. Lithium for maintenance treatment of mood disorders. Cochrane Database of Systematic Reviews 2001, Issue 3. Art. No.: CD003013. DOI: 10.1002/14651858.CD003013. **http://onlinelibrary.wiley.com/doi/10.1002/14651858.CD003013/abstract**

Macritchie K, Geddes J, Scott J, Haslam DR, Silva de Lima M, Goodwin G. Valproate for acute mood episodes in bipolar disorder. Cochrane Database of Systematic Reviews 2003, Issue 1. Art. No.: CD004052. DOI: 10.1002/14651858.CD004052. **http://onlinelibrary.wiley.com/doi/10.1002/14651858.CD004052/abstract**

Stanford School of Medicine. Stanford Self-Management Programs [Internet]. [cited 2010 Jul 22]. Available from: **http://patienteducation.stanford.edu/programs/**

Sub-Category E.7 Chronic Disease Management

Indicator E.7.2 Diabetes mellitus

Criteria	**E.7.2.1**	★	Diabetes care is based on best-practice guidelines
	E.7.2.2	❃	There is a regular medication assessment for patients with diabetes
	E.7.2.3	❃	The practice team promotes access to self-care programs and resources

Sub-Category E.7 Chronic Disease Management

Indicator E.7.2
Diabetes mellitus

Screening and care management for patients with diabetes includes shared-care with specialists and other health professionals and a system for regularly updating patients' records with lab results and other benchmarks.

Criteria:

E.7.2.1 ★ Diabetes care is based on best-practice guidelines

Interpretation

- The practice has a system for screening and managing patients with diabetes mellitus, including referrals and shared-care with specialists and allied health professionals (see also G.1.1 Continuity of Care):
  - Laboratory tests of glycemic control and positive diagnoses of diabetes are recorded in the medical record
  - There is a system to update diabetic patients' records, e.g., diabetic flow sheets, reminders on the chart, follow-ups, etc.
  - Patients are referred to dietitian services for diet management
  - See also E.1.1 Smoking Cessation, E.1.2 Alcohol, and E.1.3 Diet and Exercise
- The practice maintains a list of patients who have diabetes
- The practice undertakes an annual audit of records of patients with diabetes and has a plan to improve the results. This review includes smoking, high blood pressure, flu shot, cholesterol, prescribed medication, anticoagulation, depression, foot exam, neurological exam and referrals to other providers. It also includes the percentage of patients with diabetes mellitus who, in the past 15 months, have a record of:
  - HbA1c and the last is within optimal range
  - Blood pressure and whether it is controlled
  - Microalbuminuria (or proteinuria) and are being treated with ACE inhibitors (or A2 antagonists)
  - Serum creatinine
  - Total cholesterol, LDL and HDL and whose cholesterol is controlled
  - Referral for retinal screening
  - Foot exam
  - Depression screening
  - Presence or absence of peripheral pulses
  - Neuropathy testing
  - Being offered self-management education
  - Influenza immunization in the preceding Sept. 1 to March 31 period

Indicator E.7.2
Diabetes mellitus *(continued)*

E.7.2.2 ❋ There is a regular medication assessment for patients with diabetes

Interpretation

- The practice conducts regular medication assessments and monitors patients with diabetes (including insulin and drugs to prevent long-term complications). There is a plan to resolve any problems identified (see also D.6.2. Prescription Management)

E.7.2.3 ❋ The practice team promotes access to self-care programs and resources

Interpretation

- The practice helps patients with diabetes find local community programs, websites, pamphlets, toll-free numbers, self-care, etc.

Further Information (see up to date links at **http://quality.resources.machealth.ca**)

Canadian Diabetes Association. Canadian Diabetes Association 2013 Clinical Practice Guidelines [Internet]. 2013 [cited 2014 Jul 14]. Available from: **www.diabetes.ca/clinical-practice-education/clinical-practice-guidelines**

Stanford School of Medicine. Stanford Self-Management Programs [Internet]. [cited 2010 Jul 22]. Available from: **http://patienteducation.stanford.edu/programs/**

Sub-Category E.7 Chronic Disease Management

Indicator E.7.3 Hypertension

Criteria

E.7.3.1 ★ Hypertension management is based on best-practice guidelines

E.7.3.2 ❃ There is a regular medication assessment for patients with hypertension

E.7.3.3 ❃ The practice team promotes access to self-care programs and resources

Further Information (see up to date links at **http://quality.resources.machealth.ca**)

Canadian Hypertension Society. Home [Internet]. [cited 2010 Jul 22]. Available from: **www.hypertension.ca**

Stanford School of Medicine. Stanford Self-Management Programs [Internet]. [cited 2010 Jul 22]. Available from: **http://patienteducation.stanford.edu/programs/**

Sub-Category E.7 Chronic Disease Management

Indicator E.7.3
Hypertension

The clinical team meets best-practice guidelines for patients with hypertension, including regular medication assessments.

Criteria:

E.7.3.1 ★ Hypertension management is based on best-practice guidelines

Interpretation

- The practice management has a system for managing patients with hypertension, including referrals and shared-care with specialists and other health professionals (see G.1.1 Continuity of Care)
  - There is a system for updating the blood pressure management of patients, (e.g., flow sheets, reminders on the chart, follow-ups, etc.)
  - The practice promotes lifestyle modification (e.g., opportunistically, as part of ongoing care, other screening opportunities) to reduce the risk of high blood pressure – See E.1.1 Smoking, E.1.2 Alcohol, E.1.3 Diet and Exercise
- The practice maintains a list of patients with hypertension
- The practice undertakes an annual audit of hypertensive patients' records and has a plan to improve the results. This review includes smoking, high blood pressure, weight, flu shot, cholesterol, prescribed medication and referrals to other providers and, for example, includes the percentage of patients with hypertension:
  - Who are on hypertensive therapy
  - Who have a recent record (e.g., in the past nine months) of high blood pressure
  - Whose last blood pressure measured was controlled
  - In whom there is a record of active treatment when blood pressure levels are persistently 160/100 or higher

E.7.3.2 ✻ There is a regular medication assessment for patients with hypertension

Interpretation

- There is a regular medication assessment for patients with hypertension, and a plan to resolve any problems identified (see also D.6.2. Prescription Management)

E.7.3.3 ✻ The practice team promotes access to self-care programs and resources

Interpretation

- The practice helps patients with hypertension find local community programs, websites, pamphlets, toll-free numbers, self-care, etc.

Sub-Category E.7 Chronic Disease Management

Indicator E.7.4 Secondary prevention in coronary heart disease (CHD)

Criteria

E.7.4.1	★	CHD management is based on best-practice guidelines
E.7.4.2	❃	There is a regular medication assessment for patients with CHD
E.7.4.3	❃	The practice team promotes access to self-care programs and resources

Sub-Category E.7 Chronic Disease Management

Indicator E.7.4
Secondary prevention in coronary heart disease (CHD)

The clinical team meets the best-practice guidelines for patients with coronary heart disease (CHD), including regular medication assessments and an annual audit of care.

Criteria:

E.7.4.1 ★ CHD management is based on best-practice guidelines

Interpretation

- The practice has a system for managing patients with CHD, including referrals and shared-care with specialists and allied health workers (see G.1.1)
  - There is a system to update the CHD management of patients (e.g., flow sheets, reminders on the chart, follow-ups, etc).
  - The practice promotes lifestyle modification (e.g. opportunistically, as part of ongoing care, other screening opportunities) to reduce the risk of high blood pressure – See E.1.1 Smoking, E.1.2 Alcohol, E.1.3 Diet and Exercise
- The practice maintains a list of patients with:
  - CHD and left ventricular dysfunction
  - Atrial fibrillation
  - Newly diagnosed angina who are referred for exercise testing or specialist assessment
  - Patients discharged from hospital during the preceding three years with a diagnosis of heart attack (excluding those with a diagnosis of asthma, COPD or peripheral vascular disease)
- The practice undertakes an annual audit of CHD that includes smoking, high blood pressure, flu shot, cholesterol, atrial fibrillation, prescribed medication, anticoagulation, ACE inhibitors, echocardiogram for left ventricular dysfunction, referrals to other providers and, for example, includes the percentage of patients with CHD who, in the past 15 months, have a record of:
  - Blood pressure and whose blood pressure is controlled
  - Total cholesterol (LDL and HDL) and whose cholesterol is optimal
  - Atrial fibrillation being treated with anticoagulants (aspirin, an alternative anti-platelet therapy, or an anticoagulant) and INRs that have been recorded twice in the previous four months
  - Myocardial infarction diagnosis currently being treated with an ACE inhibitor
  - Left ventricular dysfunction confirmed by an echocardiogram and currently treated with ACE inhibitors or A2 antagonists
  - Influenza vaccination in the preceding Sept. 1–March 31 period

Indicator E.7.4
Secondary prevention in coronary heart disease (CHD) *(continued)*

E.7.4.2 ✻ There is a regular medication assessment for patients with CHD

Interpretation

- The practice has a system to regularly assess the medication of patients with CHD (aspirin, anti-coagulants, cholesterol lowering agents, beta blockers, ACE inhibitors). There is a plan to resolve problems identified (see also D.6.2 Prescription Management)

E.7.4.3 ✻ The practice team promotes access to self-care programs and resources

Interpretation

- The practice helps patients with CHD find local community programs, websites, pamphlets, toll-free numbers, self-care, etc.

Further Information (see up to date links at **http://quality.resources.machealth.ca**)

Heart and Stroke Foundation of Canada. Home [Internet]. 2010 [cited 2010 Jul 22]. Available from: **www.heartandstroke.com/site/c.ikIQLcMWJtE/b.3856593/k.B76E/For_Professionals.htm**

Institute for Clinical Systems Improvement. Health Care Guideline: Antithrombotic Therapy Supplement [Internet]. 2006 Apr [cited 2010 Jul 22]. Available from: **https://www.icsi.org/guidelines__more/catalog_guidelines_and_more/catalog_guidelines/catalog_cardiovascular_guidelines/antithrombotic/**

Stanford School of Medicine. Stanford Self-Management Programs [Internet]. [cited 2010 Jul 22]. Available from: **http://patienteducation.stanford.edu/programs/**

Sub-Category E.7 Chronic Disease Management

Indicator E.7.5 Stroke or transient ischemic attacks (TIAs)

Criteria

E.7.5.1 ★ Stroke or TIA management is based on best practices

E.7.5.2 ❋ There is a regular medication assessment for patients with stroke or TIA

E.7.5.3 ❋ The practice team promotes access to self-care programs and resources

Further Information (see up to date links at **http://quality.resources.machealth.ca**)

Heart and Stroke Foundation of Canada. Home [Internet]. 2010 [cited 2010 Jul 22]. Available from: **www.heartandstroke.ca/splash/**

Institute for Clinical Systems Improvement. Health Care Guideline: Antithrombotic Therapy Supplement [Internet]. 2006 Apr [cited 2010 Jul 22]. Available from: **https://www.icsi.org/guidelines__more/catalog_guidelines_and_more/catalog_guidelines/catalog_cardiovascular_guidelines/antithrombotic/**

Stanford School of Medicine. Stanford Self-Management Programs [Internet]. [cited 2010 Jul 22]. Available from: **http://patienteducation.stanford.edu/programs/**

Sub-Category E.7 Chronic Disease Management

Indicator E.7.5
Stroke or transient ischemic attacks (TIAs)

Best practice-guidelines for patients with stroke or transient ischemic attacks include a system for care management, regular medication assessments and an annual audit of stroke and TIA patients' records.

Criteria:

E.7.5.1 ★ Stroke or TIA management is based on best practices

Interpretation

- The practice has a system to manage patients with stroke or TIAs including referrals and shared-care with specialists and allied health professionals (see G.1.1 Continuity of Care):
  - The system includes, for example, flow sheets, reminders on the chart, follow-ups, etc.
  - The clinical team promotes lifestyle modification (e.g. opportunistically, as part of ongoing care, other screening opportunities). See E.1.1 Smoking, E.1.2 Alcohol, E.1.3 Diet and Exercise
- The practice maintains a list of patients with stroke or TIAs, identifying those with newly diagnosed strokes and TIAs who are referred for further assessment
- The practice undertakes an annual audit of stroke and TIA patients' records and has a plan to improve the results. This review includes smoking, high blood pressure, flu shot, cholesterol, atrial fibrillation, prescribed medication, anticoagulation, ACE inhibitors, echocardiogram for left ventricular dysfunction, and referrals to other providers and, for example, includes the percentage of patients with stroke or TIAs who, in the past 15 months, have a record of:
  - Confirmed diagnosis by CT or MRI scans (patients with new strokes)
  - Referral for further investigation (patients with new strokes)
  - Smoking status and whether smokers have been offered smoking-cessation advice
  - Last blood pressure of 160/90 or lower
  - Total cholesterol, HDL and LDL, and who have an optimal cholesterol
  - Treatment with anticoagulants (aspirin, an alternative anti-platelet therapy, or an anticoagulant) and INRs recorded twice in the previous four months
  - Influenza vaccination in the preceding Sept. 1-March 31 period

E.7.5.2 ❋ There is a regular medication assessment for patients with stroke or TIA

Interpretation

- The practice regularly assesses the medication of patients with stroke and TIAs (aspirin, anticoagulants, cholesterol lowering agents, anti-hypertensives). There is a plan to resolve problems identified (see also D.6.2 Prescription Management)

E.7.5.3 ❋ The practice team promotes access to self-care programs and resources

Interpretation

- The practice helps stroke or TIA patients find local community programs, websites, pamphlets, toll-free numbers, self-care, etc.

Sub-Category E.7 Chronic Disease Management

Indicator E.7.6 Asthma

Criteria

E.7.6.1	★	Asthma management is based on best-practice guidelines
E.7.6.2	❄	There is a regular medication assessment for patients with asthma
E.7.6.3	❄	The practice team promotes access to self-care programs and resources

Further Information (see up to date links at **http://quality.resources.machealth.ca**)

Canadian Thoracic Society. Guidelines and Standards - Asthma [Internet]. 2015 [cited 2015 May 19]. Available from: **www.respiratoryguidelines.ca/guideline/asthma**

Lung Association. Home [Internet]. 2010 [cited 2010 Jul 22]. Available from: **www.lung.ca/home-accueil_e.php**

Stanford School of Medicine. Stanford Self-Management Programs [Internet]. [cited 2010 Jul 22]. Available from: **http://patienteducation.stanford.edu/programs/**

Sub-Category E.7 Chronic Disease Management

Indicator E.7.6
Asthma

Best-practice guidelines for patients with asthma include a system for care management, regular medication assessments and advice on lifestyle modification.

Criteria:

E.7.6.1 ★ Asthma management is based on best-practice guidelines

Interpretation

- The practice has an evidence-based system for managing patients with asthma, including referrals and shared-care with specialists and allied health professionals (see G.1.1 Continuity of Care):
  - There is a system to update the asthma management of patients, e.g. flow sheets, reminders on the chart, follow-ups, degree of asthma control at each visit, etc.
  - The practice promotes lifestyle modification to reduce the risk of asthma, e.g. allergies, smoking (see E.1.1 Smoking)
- The practice maintains a list of patients with asthma and can identify those on asthma medications
- The practice undertakes an annual audit of asthma patients' records and has a plan to improve the results. This review includes smoking, flu shots, prescribed medications and referrals to other providers. For example, includes the percentage of patients with asthma who, in the past 15 months, have a record of:
  - Spirometry or peak flow management (for age 8 or over)
  - Smoking status (including second-hand exposure) and who have been offered smoking-cessation advice
  - Influenza vaccination in the preceding Sept. 1-March 31 period
  - Having been offered asthma-management education
  - Inhaled medication; inhaler techniques have been checked
  - Asthma relief medications
  - Asthma control medications

E.7.6.2 ❋ There is a regular medication assessment for patients with asthma

Interpretation

- The practice regularly assesses the medication of patients with asthma. There is a plan to resolve problems identified (see also D.6.2 Prescription Management)

E.7.6.3 ❋ The practice team promotes access to self-care programs and resources

Interpretation

- The practice helps asthma patients find local community programs, websites, pamphlets, toll-free numbers, self-care, etc.

Sub-Category E.7 Chronic Disease Management

Indicator E.7.7 Chronic obstructive pulmonary disease (COPD)

Criteria

E.7.7.1 ★ COPD management is based on best-practice guidelines

E.7.7.2 ❃ There is a regular medication assessment for patients with COPD

E.7.7.3 ❃ The practice team promotes access to self-care programs and resources

Further Information (see up to date links at **http://quality.resources.machealth.ca**)

Canadian Thoracic Society. Guidelines and Standards - COPD [Internet]. 2015 [cited 2015 May 19]. Available from: **www.respiratoryguidelines.ca/guideline/chronic-obstructive-pulmonary-disease**

Lung Association. Home [Internet]. 2010 [cited 2010 Jul 22]. Available from: **www.lung.ca/home-accueil_e.php**

Stanford School of Medicine. Stanford Self-Management Programs [Internet]. [cited 2010 Jul 22]. Available from: **http://patienteducation.stanford.edu/programs/**

Sub-Category E.7 Chronic Disease Management

Indicator E.7.7
Chronic obstructive pulmonary disease (COPD)

Recommended management of patients with chronic obstructive pulmonary disease includes shared-care with specialists, medication assessments and lifestyle modification advice.

Criteria:

E.7.7.1 ★ COPD management is based on best-practice guidelines
Interpretation

- The practice has a system for managing patients with COPD, including referrals and shared-care with specialists and allied health professionals (see G.1.1 Continuity of Care)
  - There is a system to update the COPD management of patients, e.g. flow sheets, reminders on the chart, follow-ups, etc.
  - The practice promotes lifestyle modification to help manage COPD and complications (see E.1.1 Smoking)
- The practice maintains a list of patients with COPD and those on COPD medication
- The practice undertakes an annual audit of COPD patients' records and has a plan to improve the results. This review includes smoking, flu shot, pneumococcal vaccination, prescribed medications, and referrals to other providers. For example, includes the percentage of patients with COPD who, in the past 15 months, have a record of:
  - Diagnosis confirmed by lung function testing
  - FEV1
  - Inhaled treatment; inhaler technique checked
  - Smoking status in the past 15 months and being offered smoking-cessation advice
  - A pneumococcus vaccine
  - Influenza vaccination in the preceding Sept. 1-March 31 period

E.7.6.2 ❋ There is a regular medication assessment for patients with COPD
Interpretation

- The practice regularly assesses the medication of patients with COPD and has a plan to resolve the problems identified (see also D.6.2 Prescription Management)

E.7.7.3 ❋ The practice team promotes access to self-care programs and resources
Interpretation

- The practice helps COPD patients find local community programs, websites, pamphlets, toll-free numbers, self-care, etc.

Sub-Category E.7 Chronic Disease Management

Indicator E.7.8 Hypothyroidism

Criteria

E.7.8.1 ★ Hypothyroidism management is based on best-practice guidelines

E.7.8.2 ❃ There is a regular medication assessment for patients with hypothyroidism

E.7.8.3 ❃ The practice team promotes access to self-care programs and resources

Sub-Category E.7 Chronic Disease Management

Indicator E.7.8
Hypothyroidism

Recommended management of patients with hypothyroidism includes shared-care with specialists and regular medication assessments.

Criteria:

E.7.8.1 ★ Hypothyroidism management is based on best-practice guidelines

Interpretation

- The practice has an evidence-based system for managing patients with hypothyroidism, including referrals and shared-care with specialists (see G.1.1)
  - There is a system to update the hypothyroidism management of patients, e.g., flow sheets, reminders on the chart, follow-ups, etc.
- The practice management maintains a list of patients with hypothyroidism and can identify those on medication
- The practice undertakes an annual audit of hypothyroidism patients' records and has a plan to improve the results. This review includes lab tests, prescribed medications and referrals to other providers, and, for example, includes the percentage of patients with hypothyroidism who, in the past 15 months, have a record of thyroid function tests and follow-up of abnormal results.

E.7.8.2 ❃ There is a regular medication assessment for patients with hypothyroidism

Interpretation

- The practice regularly assesses the medication of patients with hypothyroidism. There is a plan to resolve problems identified (see also D.6.2 Prescription Management)

E.7.8.3 ❃ The practice team promotes access to self-care programs and resources

Interpretation

- The practice helps patients with hypothyroidism find local community programs, websites, pamphlets, toll-free numbers, self-care, etc.

Further Information (see up to date links at **http://quality.resources.machealth.ca**)

Thyroid Foundation of Canada. Home [Internet]. [updated 2010 Jul 7; cited 2010 Jul 22]. Available from:**www.thyroid.ca**

GPAC: Guidelines and Protocols Advisory Committee (BC). Thyroid Function Tests in the Diagnosis and Monitoring of Adults [Internet]. 2010 Jan 1 [cited 2010 Jul 22]. Available from: **www.bcguidelines.ca/gpac/guideline_thyroid.html**

Stanford School of Medicine. Stanford Self-Management Programs [Internet]. [cited 2010 Jul 22]. Available from: **http://patienteducation.stanford.edu/programs/**

Sub-Category E.7 Chronic Disease Management

Indicator E.7.9 Epilepsy

Criteria	**E.7.9.1**	★	Epilepsy management is based on best-practice guidelines
	E.7.9.2	❄	There is a regular medication assessment for patients with epilepsy
	E.7.9.3	❄	The practice team promotes access to self-care programs and resources

Sub-Category E.7 Chronic Disease Management

Indicator E.7.9
Epilepsy

Recommended management of patients with epilepsy includes shared-care with specialists, regular medication assessments and an annual audit of patients' records.

Criteria:

E.7.9.1 ★ Epilepsy management is based on best-practice guidelines

Interpretation

- The practice has a system for managing patients with epilepsy, including referrals and shared-care with specialists (see G.1.1 Continuity of Care)
  - There is a system to update the epilepsy management of patients, e.g., flow sheets, reminders on the chart, follow-ups, etc.
- The practice maintains a list of patients with epilepsy
- The practice undertakes an annual audit of epilepsy patients' records and has a plan to improve the results. For example, this review includes lab tests, prescribed medications, referrals to other providers, and whether seizures have occurred and their frequency

E.7.9.2 ✻ There is a regular medication assessment for patients with epilepsy

Interpretation

- The practice regularly assesses the medication of patients with epilepsy and has a plan to resolve the problems identified (see also D.6.2 Prescription Management)

E.7.9.3 ✻ The practice team promotes access to self-care programs and resources

Interpretation

- The practice helps patients with epilepsy find local community programs, websites, pamphlets, toll-free numbers, self-care, etc.

Further Information (see up to date links at **http://quality.resources.machealth.ca**)

Epilepsy Ontario. Home [Internet]. [cited 2010 Jul 22].
Available from: **www.epilepsyontario.org**

Ross SD, Estok R, Chopra S, French J. Management of Newly Diagnosed Patients with Epilepsy - A Systematic Review of the Literature [Internet]. Rockville (MD): Agency for Healthcare Research and Quality (US); 2001 Sept [cited 2010 Jul 22].
Available from: **www.ncbi.nlm.nih.gov/bookshelf/br.fcgi?book=erta39**

Stanford School of Medicine. Stanford Self-Management Programs [Internet]. [cited 2010 Jul 22].
Available from: **http://patienteducation.stanford.edu/programs/**

Sub-Category E.7 Chronic Disease Management

Indicator E.7.10 Cancer

Criteria

- **E.7.10.1** ★ Cancer care (diagnosis, treatment and after-care) is based on best-practice guidelines
- **E.7.10.2** ❋ There is a regular medication assessment for patients with cancer
- **E.7.10.3** ❋ The practice team promotes access to self-care programs and resources

Further Information (see up to date links at **http://quality.resources.machealth.ca**)

Cancer Care Ontario. Home [Internet]. [updated 2010 Jul 7; cited 2010 Jul 22]. Available from: **www.cancercare.on.ca**

Cancer Care Ontario. Regional Cancer Programs [Internet]. [updated 2009 Nov 3; cited 2010 Jul 22]. Available from: **www.cancercare.on.ca/ocs/rcp/**

Memorial Sloan-Kettering Cancer Center (NY). Survivorship Care Plan [Internet]. 2010 [cited 2010 Jul 22]. Available from: **www.mskcc.org/mskcc/html/92047.cfm**

Stanford School of Medicine. Stanford Self-Management Programs [Internet]. [cited 2010 Jul 22]. Available from: **http://patienteducation.stanford.edu/programs/**

Sub-Category E.7 Chronic Disease Management

Indicator E.7.10
Cancer

Best-practice guidelines for patients with cancer include shared-care with specialists, medication assessments, and carefully maintained records of diagnosis, ongoing treatment and after-care.

Criteria:

E.7.10.1 ★ Cancer care (diagnosis, treatment and after-care) is based on best-practice guidelines

Interpretation

- The practice has an evidence-based system for managing patients with cancer, including referrals and shared-care with specialists, MRP oncologist, MRP family physician, care plans, surveillance/clinical/medication/psychosocial review reminders on the chart, etc. (see G.1.1 Continuity of Care). Some cancers require specific guidelines and care plans
  - There is a system to update the cancer management of patients, e.g., flow sheets, reminders on the chart, follow-ups, etc.
- The practice maintains a list of patients with cancer and their current disease pathway management
- The practice undertakes an annual audit of cancer patients' records and has a plan to improve the results. This review includes lab tests, prescribed medications and referrals to other providers, and, for example, includes the percentage of patients with a cancer diagnosis who:
  - Have had a visit with a member of the clinical team to review their cancer care within six months of the practice receiving notification of diagnosis
  - Are being followed by a specialist at the cancer centre (or equivalent)
  - Are being followed by the clinical team
  - Have a care plan that includes reviewing and assessing cancer treatment, surveillance, clinical examination, laboratory results, psychosocial status and medication

E.7.10.2 ❃ There is a regular medication assessment for patients with cancer

Interpretation

- The practice regularly assesses the medication of patients with cancer throughout the disease pathway management (during treatment, side-effects of chemotherapy, symptom management, ongoing and after-care medications and surveillance for adverse effects). There is a plan to resolve the problems identified (see also D.6.2 Prescription Management)

E.7.10.3 ❃ The practice team promotes access to self-care programs and resources

Interpretation

- The practice helps patients with cancer link with regional cancer programs and find local community programs, websites, pamphlets, toll-free numbers, self-care, etc.

Sub-Category E.8 Palliative Care

Indicator E.8.1 Palliative care

Criteria

- **E.8.1.1** ★ Palliative care is based on best-practice guidelines
- **E.8.1.2** ❋ There is a regular medication assessment for palliative-care patients
- **E.8.1.3** ❋ The practice team promotes access to self-care programs and resources

Further Information (see up to date links at **http://quality.resources.machealth.ca**)

College of Physicians & Surgeons of Ontario. Decision-making for the End of Life [Internet]. 2006 May/Jun/Jul [cited 2010 Jul 21].
Available from: **www.cpso.on.ca/policies/policies/default.aspx?ID=1582**

Cancer Care Ontario. Symptom Assessment & Management Tools - Edmonton Symptom Assessment (ESAS) [Internet]. [updated 2010 Apr 21; cited 2010 Jul 22].
Available from: **www.cancercare.on.ca/cms/one.aspx?objectId=58189&contextId=1377**

Stanford School of Medicine. Stanford Self-Management Programs [Internet]. [cited 2010 Jul 22].
Available from: **http://patienteducation.stanford.edu/programs/**

Sub-Category E.8 Palliative Care

Indicator E.8.1
Palliative care

Recommended management of palliative-care patients includes a system of referrals and shared-care and regular medication assessments.

Criteria:

E.8.1.1 ★ Palliative care is based on best-practice guidelines

Interpretation

- The practice has a system for managing palliative-care patients, including referral and shared-care with specialists (see G.1.1 Continuity of Care)
  - There is a system to update the management of palliative-care patients, e.g., flow sheets, reminders on the chart, follow-ups, etc.
- The practice maintains a list of palliative-care patients
- The practice undertakes an annual audit of palliative-care patients' records and has a plan to improve the results. For example, this review may assess records for live or deceased palliative patients, including: palliative-care plans, hospice-care options, pain and symptom management, family/caregiver support, mortality review, bereavement support and remembrance, as well as the percentage of patients who:
  - Have a diagnosis of palliative status
  - Have a palliative care plan
  - Died at home

E.8.1.2 ❋ There is a regular medication assessment for palliative-care patients

Interpretation

- The practice regularly assesses the medication for palliative-care patients. There is a plan to resolve the problems identified (see also D.6.2 Prescription Management)

E.8.1.3 ❋ The practice team promotes access to self-care programs and resources

Interpretation

- The practice helps palliative-care patients link with regional palliative-care programs, hospices and respite, and find local community programs, websites, ESAS, pamphlets, toll-free numbers, self-care, etc.

Sub-Category E.9 Open Indicator

Indicator E.9.1 Open indicator

Criteria

E.9.1.1 ★ ___________________________ is based on best-practice guidelines

E.9.1.2 ❋ There is a regular medication assessment for __________________

E.9.1.3 ❋ The practice team promotes access to self-care programs and resources

Sub-Category E.9 Open Indicator

Indicator E.9.1
Open Indicator

This generic indicator allows the practice team to adapt and apply the framework developed for each indicator to other clinical problems or issues identified as important and relevant to the practice.

Criteria:

E.8.1.1 ★ ____________________ is based on best-practice guidelines

Interpretation

- The practice management has an evidence-based system for managing ____________________ including referral and shared-care with specialists (see G.1.1 Continuity of Care)
  - There is a system to update the management of ____________________, e.g. flow sheets, reminders on the chart, follow-ups, etc.
- The practice maintains a list of ____________________ patients who meet the following:
- The practice management undertakes an annual audit of ________________ patients' records and has a plan to improve the results for the following:

E.8.1.2 ❋ There is a regular medication assessment for ____________________

Interpretation

- The practice regularly assesses medications for ____________. There is a plan to resolve any problems identified (see also D.6.2 Prescription Management)

E.8.1.3 ❋ The practice team promotes access to self-care programs and resources

Interpretation

- The practice helps ____________________ patients link with local community programs, and access websites, pamphlets, toll-free numbers, self-care, etc.

Further Information (see up to date links at **http://quality.resources.machealth.ca**)

For the open indicator, we suggest you search the internet for Canadian or other relevant guidelines, the Cochrane Library and other sites as required.

Stanford School of Medicine. Stanford Self-Management Programs [Internet]. [cited 2010 Jul 22]. Available from: **http://patienteducation.stanford.edu/programs/**

CATEGORY F: EFFICIENT

The indicator in this category ensures tests and reports are managed efficiently, avoiding unnecessary duplication and time wastage.

> The Institute of Medicine defines efficient as: "Avoiding waste, including waste of patient's time, equipment, supplies, ideas, and energy."

> The Ontario Health Quality Council says: "The health system should continuously look for ways to reduce waste, including waste of supplies, equipment, time, ideas and information."

Category F has 1 Sub-Category with 1 Indicator

F.1 Efficient Information Management

Indicator F.1.1
There is a system to manage patients' tests and reports efficiently

The practice has established procedures to manage patients' test results and reports, avoid duplication of tests and manage appointments efficiently.

Sub-Category F.1 Efficient Information Management

Indicator F.1.1 There is a system to manage patients' tests and reports efficiently

Criteria

F.1.1.1 ❋ The practice team has a system for avoiding duplication of tests and referrals

F.1.1.2 ❋ The practice team has a system for ensuring patients' test results are ready and available for the next appointment

F.1.1.3 ❋ The annual patient satisfaction survey asks whether the patient had unnecessary repeat testing or delays in receiving test results or consultant reports

Sub-Category F.1 Efficient Information Management

Indicator F.1.1
There is a system to manage patients' tests and reports efficiently

The practice has established procedures to manage patients' test results and reports, avoid duplication of tests and manage appointments efficiently.

Criteria:

F.1.1.1 ❋ **The practice team has a system for avoiding duplication of tests and referrals**

Interpretation

- The practice management can describe how tests and referrals are tracked to avoid duplication

F.1.1.2 ❋ **The practice team has a system for ensuring patients' test results are ready and available for the next appointment**

Interpretation

- Management can describe how the practice team ensures that test results and reports are available for the next appointment

F.1.1.3 ❋ **The annual patient satisfaction survey asks whether the patient had unnecessary repeat testing or delays in receiving test results or consultant reports**

Interpretation

- A patient satisfaction survey includes question(s) on unnecessary repeat testing and delays in receiving results or consultant reports

Further Information (see up to date links at **http://quality.resources.machealth.ca**)

White B. Preventing Errors in Your Practice: Four Principles for Better Test-Result Tracking. Fam Pract Manag [Internet]. 2002 Jul/Aug [cited 2010 Jul 22];9(7):41-44. Available from: **www.aafp.org/fpm/20020700/41four.html**

College of Physicians & Surgeons of Ontario. Medical Records [Internet]. 2006 Mar/Apr [cited 2010 Jul 21]. Available from: **www.cpso.on.ca/CPSO/media/uploadedfiles/policies/policies/policyitems/test_results.pdf?ext=.pdf**

CATEGORY G: INTEGRATED AND CONTINUOUS

Indicators in this category ensure integration and continuity of care, including services for patients with complex needs, integration with community care and provision of out-of-office care.

> The Ontario Health Quality Council says: "All parts of the health system should be organized, connected and work with one another to provide high-quality care".

Category G has 2 Sub-Categories with 3 Indicators

G.1 Continuity of Care in the Office

Indicator G.1.1

The practice team provides continuity of care

The practice team provides continuous, comprehensive and coordinated medical care, including links with hospital-based services, specialists and community-based agencies. Patients have the opportunity to develop an ongoing relationship with the practice team members.

Indicator G.1.2

The practice team provides continuity of care to patients with complex needs (high-frequency users, regular emergency users, patients often in crisis, and patients with multiple problems)

A system of alerts and management of after-hours care ensures continuous, comprehensive and coordinated medical care for patients with complex needs.

G.2 Out-of-Office Care

Indicator G.2.1

There is a policy for out-of-office care

The practice has a system to ensure patients can be treated at home, in hospital, in rehabilitation and other settings.

Sub-Category G.1 Continuity of Care in the Office

Indicator G.1.1 The practice team provides continuity of care

Criteria

G.1.1.1 ❋ The practice team supports continuity of care

G.1.1.2 ❋ Care is shared with specialists in obstetrics, psychiatry and chronic disease management

G.1.1.3 ❋ Care is integrated with other care agencies and community services

Further Information (see up to date links at **http://quality.resources.machealth.ca**)

College of Physicians & Surgeons of Ontario. Test Results Management [Internet]. 2011 Feb [cited 2015 Oct. 26]. Available from: **www.cpso.on.ca/Policies-Publications/Policy/Test-Results-Management**

Sub-Category G.1 Continuity of Care in the Office

Indicator G.1.1
The practice team provides continuity of care

The practice team provides continuous, comprehensive and coordinated medical care, including links with hospital-based services, specialists and community-based agencies. Patients have the opportunity to develop an ongoing relationship with the practice team members.

Criteria:

G.1.1.1 ❄ Continuity of care is supported by the practice team

Interpretation

- Patients attending group practices have an identified family doctor and/or other health-care professional and efforts are made to book them with their primary provider
- A range of resource people are used to support care, such as translators, sign-language interpreters, other health professionals, etc.
- A biannual audit of patient records reviews continuity of care

G.1.1.2 ❄ Care is shared with specialists in obstetrics, psychiatry and chronic disease management

Interpretation

- Clinical team members optimize shared-care with specialists
- The practice team supports patients needing long-term specialist care, such as psychiatry, obstetrics, chronic disease management and cancer care
- Incidents and complaints are reviewed and discussed and actions proposed to avoid similar problems in the future
- A biannual audit of patient records reviews shared-care with specialists

G.1.1.3 ❄ Care is integrated with other care agencies and community services

Interpretation

- The practice team links with hospital-based services, especially outpatient services
- There is a list with contact information for related community-based agencies such as CCAC, mental health services, diabetes services, palliative care, etc.
- There is a care plan system for patients referred to agencies
- Patients are provided with information about community or provincial health agencies, i.e., handouts, pamphlets or posters
- Management is knowledgeable about how the practice team communicates with other agencies and services, any barriers to communication, and how the practice has attempted to overcome those barriers

Sub-Category G.1 Continuity of Care in the Office

Indicator G.1.2 The practice team provides continuity of care to patients with complex needs (high-frequency users, regular emergency users, patients often in crisis, and patients with multiple problems)

Criteria

G.1.2.1 ★ There is a system for continuity of care for patients with complex needs

G.1.2.2 ★ There is a system for on-call/after-hours care for patients with complex needs

Sub-Category G.1 Continuity of Care in the Office

Indicator G.1.2
The practice team provides continuity of care to patients with complex needs (high-frequency users, regular emergency users, patients often in crisis, and patients with multiple problems)

A system of alerts and management of after-hours care ensures continuous, comprehensive and coordinated medical care for patients with complex needs.

Criteria:

G.1.2.1 ★ There is a system for continuity of care for patients with complex needs

Interpretation

- The practice has a list or lists of patients who have complex needs, such as mental illness, disability or terminal illness
- There is a system to alert practice team members that certain patients have special needs, e.g., red-flag notes on files or computer

G.1.2.2 ★ There is a system for on-call/after-hours care for patients with complex needs

Interpretation

- The practice has a system to ensure on-call or after-hours care of patients with complex needs

Further Information (see up to date links at **http://quality.resources.machealth.ca**)

College of Physicians & Surgeons of Ontario. Practice Tips from QA [Internet]. [cited 2010 Jul 22]. Available from: **www.cpso.on.ca/members/resources/practicepartner/practicetips/default.aspx?id=1928**

College of Physicians & Surgeons of Ontario.Test Results Management [Internet]. 2011 Feb [cited 2014 Jul 14]. Available from: **www.cpso.on.ca/CPSO/media/uploadedfiles/policies/policies/policyitems/test_results.pdf?ext=.pdf**

Chan BTB, Ovens HJ. Frequent users of emergency departments: Do they also use family physicians' services? Can Fam Physician [Internet]. 2002 Oct [cited 2010 Jul 22];48:1654-1660. Available from: **www.cfp.ca/cgi/reprint/48/10/1654.pdf**

Ontario Association of Community Care Access Centres. Map services near you [Internet]. [cited 2014 Jul 14]. Available from: **http://healthcareathome.ca/**

Many communities produce resources about agencies and institutions:

Hamilton Academy of Medicine. Home [Internet]. 2010 [cited 2010 Jul 22]. Available from: **www.hamiltondoctors.ca/**

Findhelp Information Services. Blue Book of Community Services (Toronto) [Internet]. [cited 2010 Jul 22]. Available from: **www.211toronto.ca/index.jsp**

Sub-Category G.2 Out-of-Office Care

Indicator G.2.1 There is a policy for out-of-office care

Criteria

G.2.1.1 ❋ The clinical team provides house calls to patients who require them

G.2.1.2 ❋ The practice team has a system to keep track of and manage patients who are in hospital, rehabilitation or other settings

Sub-Category G.2 Out-of-Office Care

Indicator G.2.1
There is a policy for out-of-office care

The practice has a system to ensure patients can be treated at home, in hospital, in rehabilitation and other settings.

Criteria:

G.2.1.1 ❋ The clinical team provides house calls to patients who require them

Interpretation

- The practice has a list of patients who are routinely seen at home
- There is a system to manage patients requiring house calls (including reminders to visit, charting, billing and links with other agencies providing care in the home)

G.2.1.2 ❋ The practice team has a system to keep track of and manage patients who are in hospital, rehabilitation or other settings

Interpretation

- The practice has a system for tracking, visiting, managing and transferring patients to hospitals, rehabilitation centres and other settings
- Visits are recorded in the charts and billed
- An annual audit includes a review of the records of patients who are in hospital, rehabilitation and other settings

Further Information (see up to date links at **http://quality.resources.machealth.ca**)

Ontario Association of Community Care Access Centres. Main Page [Internet]. [cited 2010 Jul 22]. Available from: **http://oaccac.on.ca/**

CATEGORY H: APPROPRIATE PRACTICE RESOURCES

Indicators in this category include human resources management, physical facilities, workplace safety and fire management, and practice improvement and planning.

> The Ontario Health Quality Council defines appropriate resources in this way: "The health system should have enough qualified providers, funding, information, equipment, supplies and facilities to look after people's health needs."

Category H has 4 Sub-Categories with 11 Indicators

H.1 Human Resources Management

Indicator H.1.1
All clinical team members of the practice are qualified and certified
Clinical team members are qualified and certified, and maintain updated licences, credentials and privileges.

Indicator H.1.2
The practice team has human resources policies and procedures
The practice has human resources policies and procedures, including documented workplace policies and signed employment contracts for each practice member.

Indicator H.1.3
The practice members function as a team
The practice members function as a team; regular practice meetings are provided and recorded.

Indicator H.1.4
The practice team members balance work and home life
The practice team members balance work and home life; part-time and flexible work hours are supported, and parental needs incorporated into planning.

H.2 Physical Facilities

Indicator H.2.1
The practice is physically accessible
The practice is physically accessible to most patients, including those with mobility problems.

Indicator H.2.2
The practice's waiting area accommodates patients and their family members
Recommendations for the waiting area include four seats per FTE doctor, and room to accommodate guide dogs and mobility scooters.

Indicator H.2.3
Examination areas ensure patient comfort and privacy
Each examination room is comfortable and private; conversations cannot be overheard.

H.3 Workplace Safety and Fire Management

Indicator H.3.1
The practice is committed to workplace safety
The practice provides a safe working environment and complies with all WSIB and OHSA requirements.

Indicator H.3.2
Fire risk is minimized
Recommendations for fire safety include an approved evacuation plan and appropriate fire protection equipment.

H.4 Practice Improvement and Planning

Indicator H.4.1
The practice team promotes continuous quality improvement (CQI)
There is a designated person responsible for ensuring the practice team promotes a culture of continuous quality improvement (CQI).

Indicator H.4.2
The practice team has a formulated practice plan for improvement and risk management
The practice team undertakes regular purposeful planning for improvement and risk management, including disaster planning.

Sub-Category H.1 Human Resources

Indicator H.1.1 All clinical team members of the practice are qualified and certified

Criteria

H.1.1.1 ★ The clinical team members maintain updated licences, registration, certification, maintenance of certification, and medical protective insurance (CMPA or equivalent)

H.1.1.2 ★ The clinical team members maintain updated credentials and privileges for procedures, prescribing, medical directives, etc.

Sub-Category H.1 Human Resources

Indicator H.1.1
All clinical team members of the practice are qualified and certified

Clinical team members are qualified and certified, and maintain updated licences, credentials and privileges.

Criteria

H.1.1.1 ★ The clinical team members maintain updated licences, registration, certification, maintenance of certification, and medical protective insurance (CMPA or equivalent)

Interpretation

- The practice management maintains a record, updated annually, of team members' licences, qualifications and certifications

H.1.1.2 ★ The clinical team members maintain updated credentials and privileges for procedures, prescribing, medical directives etc.

Interpretation

- The practice has an annually reviewed list of those who have the credentials and privileges to perform procedures, prescribing, medical directives, etc.

Further Information (see up to date links at **http://quality.resources.machealth.ca**)

(Licensing, maintenance of licences and insurance apply to all health disciplines. The following are examples for family physicians and nurse practitioners.)

College of Physicians & Surgeons of Ontario. Annual Membership Renewal [Internet]. 2010 [cited 2010 Jul 20]. Available from: **www.cpso.on.ca/members/membership/default.aspx?id=1874**

College of Family Physicians of Canada. Mainpro© – Maintenance of Proficiency [Internet]. 2010 [updated 2010 Jun 10; cited 2010 Jul 20]. Available from: **www.cfpc.ca/mainpro/**

Canadian medical Protectivce Association. Shared care: issues you should consider [Internet]. 2005 Jun [updated 2008 May; cited 2014 Jul 14].
Available from: **https://oplfrpd5.cmpa-acpm.ca/en/web/guest/-/shared-care-issues-you-should-consider**

Canadian Medical Protective Association & Canadian Nurses Protective Society. CMPA/CNPS Joint Statement on Liability Protection for Nurse Practitioners and Physicians in Collaborative Practice [Internet]. 2005 Mar [cited 2015 Oct 08]. Available from: **www.cnps.ca/index.php?page=29**

Canadian Nurses Association, Canadian Medical Association & Canadian Pharmacists Association. Joint Position Statement – Scopes of Practice [Internet]. 2003 Apr [cited 2014 Jul 14].
Available from: **www.cna-aiic.ca/~/media/cna/page-content/pdf-en/10%20-%20ps66_scopes_of_practice_june_2003_e.pdf**

Sub-Category H.1 Human Resources

Indicator H.1.2 The practice has human resources policies and procedures

Criteria

H.1.2.1	★	The practice has documented workplace policies, including recruitment, retention and appointment criteria, and disciplinary procedures
H.1.2.2	★	There are written and signed employment contracts with terms and conditions for each practice member
H.1.2.3	★	All members of the practice team have job descriptions that include key tasks, reporting relationships and annual review dates.
H.1.1.4	★	All members of the practice team have been oriented and trained in procedures relevant to their position
H.1.2.5	❃	Performance reviews are conducted annually for all practice team members, including practice partners
H.1.2.6	❃	The practice supports continuous professional development (CPD)
H.1.2.7	★	The practice has a policy and procedure for financial management

Sub-Category H.1 Human Resources

Indicator H.1.2
The practice has human resources policies and procedures

The practice has human resources policies and procedures, including documented workplace policies and signed employment contracts for each practice member.

Criteria

H.1.2.1 ★ The practice has documented workplace policies, including recruitment, retention and appointment criteria, and disciplinary procedures

Interpretation

- The practice has an office procedures manual covering the practice's administrative policies and procedures; the staff have access to this manual
- The practice management has clearly stated workplace policies, including explicit processes for the recruitment and selection of staff

H.1.2.2 ★ There are written and signed employment contracts with terms and conditions for each practice member

Interpretation

- The practice management has a system for maintaining employment contracts (signed with terms and conditions for each practice member, including locums)

H.1.2.3 ★ All members of the practice team have job descriptions that include key tasks, reporting relationships and annual review dates

Interpretation

- The practice management can produce current job descriptions of all team members, including key tasks, functional relationships and annual review dates

H.1.2.4 ★ All members of the practice team have been oriented and trained in procedures relevant to their position

Interpretation

- There is an orientation manual for new practice-team members, including temporary staff and locums
- The practice management ensures and records staff orientation

H.1.2.5 ❃ Performance reviews are conducted annually for all practice-team members, including practice partners

Interpretation

- The practice management has a system for performance reviews that includes due dates for reviews, actual dates of reviews, outcomes and plans (including plans for continuous professional development, CPD)

Indicator H.1.2
The practice has human resources policies and procedures *(continued)*

H.1.2.6 ✻ The practice supports continuous professional development (CPD)

Interpretation

- The practice management ensures:
  - Practice team members identify CPD learning needs as part of their annual review
  - CPD activities are supported (with money, time, or equivalent)
  - A range of educational resources and materials are available to members of the practice for reference purposes (internet access, books, journals, etc.)

H.1.2.7 ★ The practice has a policy and procedure for financial management

Interpretation

- The practice management has:
  - A policy for handling financial transactions
  - A list of people who have defined levels of responsibility for finances
  - An annual accounting audit review of financial procedures and transactions

Further Information (see up to date links at **http://quality.resources.machealth.ca**)

Ministry of Health & Long-Term Care (Ontario). Family Health Teams – Advancing Primary Health Care: Guide to Collaborative Practice [Internet]. 2005 Jun 4. [cited 2014 Jul 14]. Available from: **www.health.gov.on.ca/en/pro/programs/fht/docs/fht_collab_team.pdf**

College of Family Physicians of Canada. Mainpro© – Maintenance of Proficiency [Internet]. 2010 [updated 2010 Jun 10; cited 2010 Jul 20]. Available from: **www.cfpc.ca/mainpro/**

McNamara C. Basic Guide to Financial Management in For-Profits [Internet]. [cited 2010 Jul 19]. Available from: **http://managementhelp.org/businessfinance/index.htm**

Sub-Category H.1 Human Resources

Indicator H.1.3 The practice members function as a team

Criteria

H.1.3.1 ❋ The practice promotes team functioning activities

H.1.3.2 ❋ The practice team evaluates team functioning

Sub-Category H.1 Human Resources

Indicator H.1.3
The practice members function as a team

The practice members function as a team; regular practice meetings are provided and recorded.

Criteria

H.1.3.1 ❋ The practice promotes team functioning activities

Interpretation

- The practice management:
  - Knows how the practice team responds to new needs, communicates routinely and manages challenges
  - Can produce a record of regular practice meetings and action-oriented minutes
  - Can produce a record of extraordinary meetings and their minutes
  - Ensures all members of the practice team have the opportunity to participate in planning and decision-making
  - Provides multidisciplinary events for team members (training, social, etc.)
  - Recognizes the contributions of practice team members

H.1.3.2 ❋ The practice team evaluates team functioning

Interpretation

- Management can describe how the practice team undertakes formal and informal evaluation of team functioning

Further Information (see up to date links at **http://quality.resources.machealth.ca**)

Way D, Jones L, Baskerville B, Busing N. Primary health care services provided by nurse practitioners and family physicians in shared practice. CMAJ [Internet]. 2001 October 30 [cited 2010 Jul 21];165(9):1210-1214. Available from: **www.ncbi.nlm.nih.gov/pmc/articles/PMC81583/**

Ministry of Health & Long-Term Care (Ontario). Family Health Teams – Advancing Primary Health Care: Guide to Collaborative Practice [Internet]. 2005 Jun 4. [cited 2014 Jul 14]. Available from: **www.health.gov.on.ca/en/pro/programs/fht/docs/fht_collab_team.pdf**

Sub-Category H.1 Human Resources

Indicator H.1.4 The practice team members balance work and home life

Criteria H.1.4.1 ❋ The practice supports a healthy balance between work and home life

Sub-Category H.1 Human Resources

Indicator H.1.4
The practice team members balance work and home life

The practice team members balance work and home life; part-time and flexible work hours are supported, and parental needs incorporated into planning.

Criteria

H.1.4.1 ✻ The practice supports a healthy balance between work and home life

Interpretation

- The practice management:
  - Supports part-time hours and flexible work hours when appropriate
  - Incorporates parental needs into workday planning
  - Ensures working hours and staffing arrangements balance the needs of patients and caregivers (early hours, evening hours)
- The practice management can produce:
  - A human resources manual that includes descriptions for vacation, lieu time, sick leave, CPD time, leave of absence, sabbatical, maternity leave, paternity leave, etc.
  - A practice team satisfaction survey, including how issues were resolved

Further Information (see up to date links at **http://quality.resources.machealth.ca**)

Physician Health Program & Professionals Health Program (OMA). PHP – Home [Internet]. 2009 [cited 2015 May 19]. Available from: **http://php.oma.org/index.htm**

Ministry of Health & Long-Term Care (Ontario). Family Health Teams – Advancing Primary Health Care: Guide to Collaborative Practice [Internet]. 2005 Jun 4. [cited 2014 Jul 14]. Available from: **www.health.gov.on.ca/en/pro/programs/fht/docs/fht_collab_team.pdf**

Sub-Category H.2 Physical Facilities

Indicator H.2.1 The practice is physically accessible

Criteria

- **H.2.1.1** ❋ Practice signs are clear, visible and placed so they can be read from a distance
- **H.2.1.2** ❋ Most people with mobility problems can access the practice
- **H.2.1.3** ❋ There is adequate parking close to the practice

Sub-Category H.2 Physical Facilities

Indicator H.2.1
The practice is physically accessible

The practice is physically accessible to most patients, including those with mobility problems.

Criteria

H.2.1.1 ✻ Practice signs are clear, visible and placed so they can be read from a distance

Interpretation

- The practice signs are clear and can be read without difficulty from a distance, including directions for patients (e.g., toilets, reception, exit signs, fire extinguishers)
- The practice undertakes an annual patient satisfaction questionnaire that includes questions about physical access, and records follow-up to feedback suggestions

H.2.1.2 ✻ Most people with mobility problems can access the practice

Interpretation

- There are aids to ensure access to the clinic, such as railings, ramps, lifts, wheelchair access, toilet supports, chairs with armrests, steps beside examining couches, easy-opening entrance doors and a bell to call for assistance
- There should be room for patients awaiting consultation to manoeuvre wheelchairs and park mobility scooters in the practice without blocking access.
- The practice management can list the number of off-site visits to patients unable to access the physical premises

H.2.1.3 ✻ There is adequate parking close to the practice

Interpretation

- The practice has sufficient parking for patients
- Disabled parking spaces are located close to the entrance of the practice

Further Information (see up to date links at **http://quality.resources.machealth.ca**)

Ontario Human Rights Commission. Disability and the Duty to Accommodate: Your Rights and Responsibilities [Internet]. 2008 [updated 2010 Jul 20; cited 2010 Jul 21].
Available from: **www.ohrc.on.ca/en/issues/disability**

Ontario Human Rights Commission. Submission of the Ontario Human Rights Commission: Concerning Barrier-Free Access Requirements in the Ontario Building Code [Internet]. 2002 Mar 1 [cited 2010 Jul 21]. Available from: **www.ohrc.on.ca/en/submission-ontario-human-rights-commission-concerning-barrier-free-access-requirements-ontario**

College of Physicians & Surgeons of Ontario. Physicians and the Ontario Human Rights Code [Internet]. 2008 Dec [cited 2010 Jul 21]. Available from: **www.cpso.on.ca/policies/policies/default.aspx?ID=2102**

Sub-Category H.2 Physical Facilities

Indicator H.2.2 The practice's waiting area accommodates patients and their family members

Criteria	**H.2.2.1**	★	The waiting area meets the needs of patients
	H.2.2.2	❃	The waiting area meets the needs of children
	H.2.2.3	❃	The waiting area has current materials

Sub-Category H.2 Physical Facilities

Indicator H.2.2
The practice's waiting area accommodates patients and their family members

Recommendations for the waiting area include four seats per FTE doctor, and room to accommodate guide dogs and mobility scooters.

Criteria

H.2.2.1 ★ The waiting area meets the needs of patients

Interpretation

- Four seats per FTE doctor are recommended
- The temperature year-round should be comfortable
- The waiting room should accommodate guide dogs comfortably – guide dogs are trained to lie at the handler's feet and there should be space for them away from foot traffic areas and doorways
- The seats have a range of heights and arm supports to assist patients with disabilities such as arthritis or hip problems
- There is an area for parking mobility scooters

H.2.2.2 ❃ The waiting area meets the needs of children

Interpretation

- There is a children's space
- Toys should be safe for all ages
- Toys should be cleaned regularly
- Safety hazards should be eliminated, e.g., electric sockets have safety plugs, electrical cords are stowed, stairs have barriers, etc.
- Parenting information in the waiting area adheres to the Child Friendly Office and Baby-Friendly standards

H.2.2.3 ❃ The waiting area has current materials

Interpretation

- Magazines are placed at a suitable height for disabled people
- Reading materials and posters are current
- Patients can access relevant health information (brochures, computers, video/audio recordings, etc.)

Further Information (see up to date links at **http://quality.resources.machealth.ca**)

Sub-Category H.2 Physical Facilities

Indicator H.2.3 Examination areas ensure patients' comfort and privacy

Criteria **H.2.3.1** ★ Each examination room is comfortable and private

Sub-Category H.2 Physical Facilities

Indicator H.2.3
Examination areas ensure patients' comfort and privacy

Each examination room is comfortable and private; conversations cannot be overheard.

Criteria

H.2.3.1 ★ Each examination room is comfortable and private

Interpretation

- The examination areas are private
- The examination room is kept at a comfortable temperature for patients who need to undress
- There is good lighting for all examinations
- The examination room is not affected by noise that interferes with the patient-doctor visit (e.g., traffic, radio, practice team conversations, etc.)
- Patient visits cannot be heard by people in the waiting room or other areas of the practice
- Examination couches are at a safe height or have portable steps available

Further Information (see up to date links at **http://quality.resources.machealth.ca**)

College of Physicians & Surgeons of Ontario. A Practical Guide for Safe and Effective Office Based Practices [Internet]. 2009 Apr [cited 2014 Jul 14].
Available from: **www.cpso.on.ca/uploadedFiles/policies/guidelines/office/Safe-Practices.pdf**

Sub-Category H.3 Workplace Safety and Fire Management

Indicator H.3.1 The practice is committed to workplace safety

Criteria

H.3.1.1 ⚖ The practice team complies with Workplace Safety and Insurance Board policies and identifies and manages WSIB procedures

H.3.1.2 ⚖ The practice team complies with the Occupational Health and Safety Act (OHSA)

H.3.1.3 ⚖ There is a record of screening and immunization status for all members of the practice team

Further Information (see up to date links at **http://quality.resources.machealth.ca**)

Workplace Safety and Insurance Board (Ontario). Your Health and Safety Rights and Responsibilities [Internet]. [cited 2010 Jul 21].
Available from: **www.wsib.on.ca/en/community/WSIB/230/ArticleDetail/24338?vgnextoid=6c44e35c819d7210VgnVCM100000449c710aRCRD**

Workplace Safety and Insurance Board (Ontario). Employer's Report of Injury/Disease (Form 7) [Internet]. [cited 2010 Jul 21].
Available from: **www.wsib.on.ca/en/community/WSIB/230/ArticleDetail/24338?vgnextoid=5937ab84c59d7210VgnVCM100000449c710aRCRD**

Workplace Safety and Insurance Board (Ontario). "In Case of Injury at Work" Poster (Form 82) [Internet]. [cited 2010 Jul 21].
Available from: **www.wsib.on.ca/en/community/WSIB/230/ArticleDetail/24338?vgnextoid=cafee35c819d7210VgnVCM100000449c710aRCRD**

Ministry of Labour (Ontario). Preventing Workplace Violence And Workplace Harassment [Internet]. [updated 2010 Jun 15; cited 2010 Jul 21].
Available from: **www.labour.gov.on.ca/english/hs/sawo/pubs/fs_workplaceviolence.php**

Workplace Safety and Insurance Board (Ontario). Making Ergonomics Work [Internet]. [cited 2010 Jul 21].
Available from: **http://batikyogya.files.wordpress.com/2007/07/ergonomics.pdf**

Association of Canadian Ergonomists. ACE Website [Internet]. [cited 2010 Jul 21].
Available from: **www.ace-ergocanada.ca/index.php?lang=en**

Canadian Centre for Occupational Health and Safety. OSH Answers: Ergonomics [Internet]. [cited 2010 Jul 21].
Available from: **www.ccohs.ca/oshanswers/ergonomics/**

Occupational Health Clinics for Ontario Workers. Occupational Health Clinics for Ontario Workers Inc. [Internet]. 2003 [cited 2010 Jul 21].
Available from: **www.ohcow.on.ca**

Sub-Category H.3 Workplace Safety and Fire Management

Indicator H.3.1
The practice is committed to workplace safety

The practice provides a safe working environment and complies with all WSIB and OHSA requirements.

Criteria

H.3.1.1 ⚖ The practice team complies with Workplace Safety and Insurance Board policies and identifies and manages WSIB procedures

Interpretation

- The practice management can produce:
  - The WSIB Manual and a policy that describes how the practice meets health and safety legislation
  - A list of events, actions and training in WSIB issues
  - The log of WSIB meetings and minutes taken at the meetings (including how the team is made aware of additions or alterations to WSIB procedures)
  - The WSIB accident and incidents list (completed incident forms – Form 7 – must be retained on file in the practice)
- Management can identify the WSIB officer responsible for WSIB in the practice
- The practice management can describe how the practice team implements ergonomic workstations, smoke-free workplaces and bio-medically safe workplaces

H.3.1.2 ⚖ The practice team complies with the Occupational Health and Safety Act (OHSA)

Interpretation

- The practice complies with the OHSA with respect to violence and harassment in the workplace.

H.3.1.3 ⚖ There is a record of screening and immunization status for all members of the practice team

Interpretation

- The practice maintains a record of the immunization status for all practice team members (hepatitis B and C, TB, measles, rubella, polio, influenza, tetanus, diphtheria and pneumococcus)
- The practice has a prompt and organized process to manage exposure to blood and body fluids such as needle-stick injuries (see D.4.1.3)

Sub-Category H.3 Workplace Safety and Fire Management

Indicator H.3.2 Fire risk is minimized

Criteria H.3.2.1 ⚖ The practice team has a fire-management plan

Sub-Category H.3 Workplace Safety and Fire Management

Indicator H.3.2
Fire risk is minimized

Recommendations for fire safety include an approved evacuation plan and appropriate fire-protection equipment.

Criteria

H.3.2.1 ⚖ The practice team has a fire-management plan

Interpretation

- The practice management can produce:
  - An evacuation plan approved by the Ontario Fire Marshal
  - The Fire and Emergency Code of Practice
  - The results of the six monthly audits that have been undertaken in accordance with the Fire and Emergency Code of practice, including fire drills and the regular audit of fire protection equipment (e.g., smoke alarms, CO alarms, fire extinguishers, paper chart protection and electronic back-ups for patient record management)
- The practice management can identify the fire warden and deputy

Further Information (see up to date links at **http://quality.resources.machealth.ca**)

Ministry of Municipal Affairs and Housing (Ontario). Ontario Building Code [Internet]. 2002 [updated 2010 Jul 15; cited 2010 Jul 21].
Available from: **www.obc.mah.gov.on.ca/**

Building Code Act (Ontario): Section 3.7.5 Health Care Facility Systems [Internet]. 2010 Apr 1 [cited 2010 Jul 21]. Available from: **www.publications.serviceontario.ca/ecomlinks/BuildingCodeUpdate.pdf**

Office of the Fire Marshal (Ontario). The Fire Protection and Prevention Act, 1997 and the Ontario Fire Code [Internet]. [updated 2010 Feb 17; cited 2010 Jul 21].
Available from: **www.e-laws.gov.on.ca/html/statutes/english/elaws_statutes_97f04_e.htm**

Office of the Fire Marshal (Ontario). Home [Internet]. [updated 2014 Jun 25; cited 2014 Jul 14].
Available from: **www.mcscs.jus.gov.on.ca/english/FireMarshal/OFMLanding/OFM_main.html**

Office of the Fire Marshal (Ontario). Guidelines: Fire Drills [Internet]. 2004 Oct [updated 2010 Feb 17; cited 2014 Jul 14].
Available from: **www.mcscs.jus.gov.on.ca/stellent/groups/public/@mcscs/@www/@ofm/documents/webasset/ecofm000489.pdf**

Sub-Category H.4 Practice Improvement and Planning

Indicator H.4.1 The practice team promotes continuous quality improvement (CQI)

Criteria

H.4.1.1 ❋ The practice team has a CQI plan

H.4.1.2 ❋ There is a designated person responsible for coordinating CQI activities

Sub-Category H.4 Practice Improvement and Planning

Indicator H.4.1
The practice team promotes continuous quality improvement (CQI)

There is a designated person responsible for ensuring the practice team promotes a culture of continuous quality improvement (CQI).

Criteria

H.4.1.1 ✻ **The practice team has a CQI plan**

Interpretation

- Management can produce:
  - The CQI plan and PDSA cycles for the next year
  - The list of CQI activities undertaken in the past year

H.4.1.2 ✻ **There is a designated person responsible for coordinating CQI activities**

Interpretation

- The practice management can identify the person responsible for CQI activities

Further Information (see up to date links at **http://quality.resources.machealth.ca**)

Institute for Healthcare Improvement. Plan-Do-Study-Act (PDSA) Worksheet (IHI Tool) [Internet]. [cited 2010 Jul 21].
Available from: **www.ihi.org/IHI/Topics/Improvement/ImprovementMethods/Tools/Plan-Do-Study-Act+(PDSA)+Worksheet.htm**

Quality Improvement & Innovation Partnership (Ontario). Home [Internet]. 2010 [cited 2010 Jul 21].
Available from: **www.ohpe.ca/node/10430**

Sub-Category H.4 Practice Improvement and Planning

Indicator H.4.2 The practice team has a formulated practice plan for improvement and risk management

Criteria

H.4.2.1 ❋ The practice team has a five-year practice improvement plan

H.4.2.2 ❋ There is a disaster plan

H.4.2.3 ❋ There is a pandemic plan

Sub-Category H.4 Practice Improvement and Planning

Indicator H.4.2
The practice team has a formulated practice plan for improvement and risk management

The practice team undertakes regular purposeful planning for improvement and risk management, including disaster planning.

Criteria

H.4.2.1 ❋ **The practice team has a five-year practice improvement plan**

Interpretation

- The practice has a current five-year practice improvement plan that:
  - Is reviewed every year (and an annual business plan prepared)
  - Encourages input from all team members
  - Encourages patients' input

H.4.2.2 ❋ **There is a disaster plan**

Interpretation

- The current disaster plan covers:
  - Practice-specific disasters such as armed robbery, power failure, computer hardware/software failure, and fire
  - Local emergencies such as multiple victim accidents, bio-hazards exposure, air disasters, etc.
  - Natural disasters such as earthquakes and floods, etc.

H.4.2.3 ❋ **There is a pandemic plan**

Interpretation

- The practice's pandemic plan includes:
  - Local preparation for flu/infectious pandemics
  - Collaboration with local public health and other primary care providers

Further Information (see up to date links at **http://quality.resources.machealth.ca**)

Ministry of Health & Long-Term Care (Ontario). Emergency Planning and Preparedness [Internet], [updated 2010 Apr 22; cited 2010 Jul 21]. Available from: **www.health.gov.on.ca/english/providers/program/emu/emu_mn.html**

Ministry of Health & Long-Term Care (Ontario). Influenza Pandemic – Ministry Programs[Internet]. 2008 [updated 2010 Apr 22; cited 2010 Jul 21]. Available from: **www.health.gov.on.ca/en/public/programs/emu/pan_flu/**

San Francisco Department of Public Health. Clinic/Office Disaster and Emergency Planning [Internet]. 2008 Jul [cited 2015 Oct 08]. Available from: **www.sfcdcp.org/document.html?id=309.**

CPSIA information can be obtained at www.ICGtesting.com
Printed in the USA
LVIW01n0932051016
507478LV00001B/1